SIX MO

to say g

Six months to say goodbye

When a son took care of his mum during that precious time.

A true story
by Lee Hayward

Hayward, Lee D

Six months to say goodbye:
When a son cared for his mum during that precious time

Lee D. Hayward. – 2nd ed.

Paperback ISBN: 0 – 9748643 – 1– 5

I.   Title

SECOND PAPER BACK EDITION

This book is dedicated with love and precious memories to:

Tina Hayward ("Mum")
Your life touched so many hearts,
and to the many special friends that touched yours;
especially (for sharing your time with mum,
for your warmth and encouragement)
Minnie & Mark, Mike & Sam,
Norma & family, Leanne,
Adrian & Laura and Nicky.

CONTENTS

CONTENTS (continued)

I believe in the sun
even when
it is not shining.

I believe in love
even when
I cannot feel it.

I believe in God
even when
He is silent.

(written on a wall by
Jewish prisoners in Cologne)

Acknowledgements

I thank Mum for sharing with me and teaching me so much about the good in life and in people (this has enabled me to move forward in life when there is so much that could have held me back); for enrichment, encouragement and an enduring strength of spirit, and for impressing upon me that there is so much more to life than just things.

I am sincerely grateful to the true friends in my life for their encouragement, love and support including Nicky Smith for her kindness and strength during the writing of this book, for her patient editing skills throughout the duration of this project, I am so grateful to you. Also Mike, Becky and young Mike Speer for all their love and care and for being my "family" in the U.S.; Don & Nancy Conwell, Dr. Bala & Ann Rao and my good friend Craig Glenzer.

Charlie Back has been there during many times I needed kind words, and practical help. I owe many thanks to Jay Briggle for his friendship and numerous suggestions concerning this book.

Bob & Peggy Saxon, Bob was tremendous in taking the time to run through the early drafts giving much input and doing the initial editing.

I am so grateful as well, to so many that looked over the initial drafts, for their honest feed back, enabling me to see the emerging book through the readers eyes. Their words have been of great encouragement. They include Sherrie & Keith Ferstl, who spent hours of their precious time poring over the manuscript, making careful and caring suggestions; Tim Gregory, Sharon McIntosh-Ryan, Sheila, Glenn & Kim McGorty and Edie Seeton.

Many thanks are also due to Erwig Martinez for his input of ideas into the early design for the book cover and Jason Parish for his skilful photography and graphic designing of the front cover and back insert picture as well as all your time and effort to make it the great cover it is today.

Finally, a tremendous debt of gratitude was earned by the staff and nurses at the BRI (Bristol Royal Infirmary) and Frenchay Hospitals, St. Peter's Hospice and St. Monica's and district nurses, doctors and staff at Western College Medical Practice, Bristol; for the care, love and dedication they showed in their work and towards Mum. I could never say enough in praise of the many angels who did so much to help Mum in those final months. Thank you.

~ ⚓ ~

<u>Six months to say goodbye</u>

The Doctor said, "I'm sorry. She only has six months to live."

This is the true story of a son and his mum, their adventures and travels and how, in the course of time, their roles were suddenly reversed.

I was fortunate enough to be able to be with her and care for her throughout that special time, and our final journey

Tina Hayward: November 7, 1937 – June 10, 2002. The most important thing here is that little "dash" between the dates; it represents a lifetime. It may not look like much, but what we do with that "dash" is what counts. Mum did a lot with her dash.

I hope this book will be an encouragement to those who are about to embark on this type of journey, a comfort for those in the process, and an unspoken bonding with those who have already been there and come back.

Introduction

So much of where we are in life today is the result of a series of choices we've made in the past. There will always be choices and the most we can hope to do is to choose the best way forward, using wisdom and discernment where we can. Our circumstances, of course, often affect the decisions that we make. I was in circumstances that, thankfully, made it quite possible for me to return to England in the manner that I did, and fulfill the choice I made. The sacrifices didn't directly affect anyone else but me, which may not be the case for everyone. If there is a choice, and you are able to, sleep on it and pray about it. Looking back, the joy and peace on my mum's face was a greater reward than anything else I could have received.

When our lives get interrupted, as they often do, we somehow take care of the situation that has arisen and then pick up our routine where we left off. Sometimes we ignore the interruption and carry on, more aware of our own needs than those of others; perhaps we are just too busy? However, when the situation involves a loved one, we are inclined to drop whatever we are doing and go to the other's aid. There are numerous situations where certain types of illness and circumstances make it no longer possible for our loved one to be cared for at home. There are times when the patient deteriorates to a point where it is simply unbearable to see him or her in that condition any longer. At these times, it is the love between two people that can transcend the circumstances in which they find themselves and transform a sterile ward cubicle (for example) into an intimate and friendly environment.

Given the choice, we will go to extraordinary lengths to be there, wherever "there" might be. We often hear about circumstances where complete strangers go to great lengths, even risking their own lives, to help or rescue others and regularly witness this selfless dedication in members of our police forces, fire departments, search & rescue teams, armed forces and the medical profession. Sometimes quite ordinary people happen to be around at the precise moment when someone desperately needs help. There are many unknown heroes we never hear about who have made a real difference in another's life.

We are all someone's hero - or at least we could be... If you are about to care for, presently do or have already taken care of a loved one, make no mistake about it - you are a hero to that person.

The sacrifices, dedication and commitment, often in difficult and emotional situations, will have been immensely valued by family and friends, even if in some situations the one being cared about is unaware of your love, concern and care. Perhaps you are the only one who knows what you went through to do the kind thing you did? Be assured your life is richer and your spirit stronger because of what you gave, or will be through what you are giving.

May the light you shine brighten the path for one whose own glows dimmer.

Lee Hayward

Chapter 1

Mum

Fatima Carim was born in Johannesburg, South Africa, towards the end of 1937. Her father came from a well-to-do Indian family and was a successful businessman. He disappointed his family when he eloped with the Malaysian house servant. She later became my mother's mum. Fatima (Mum) was the first of six children, all girls. They lived in Johannesburg until she was seven years old. Due to his growing fear of apartheid rule and all the pain and suffering that could come along with it, her father, in 1942, moved the family, the contents of the house and all the bags they could carry to India by passenger ship.

They arrived in Bombay and took a train to Delhi. They moved into a big two-storey farmhouse. Mr. Carim grew and sold vegetables and other food, wholesale and retail. The family had servants in the home and workers to work the fields. Five years later, serious difficulties came to a head between various religious factions. In 1947, the British were about to leave, giving India self rule (I don't think they could stand anymore English food!). At the time, Mum's family had a great deal more than the "have-nots." The "have-nots" wanted to have what people in their situation had, and all indications pointed to complete civil unrest once the British were gone. Anticipating the probable loss of all property, and very likely their lives, Mum's father decided to uproot the entire family again and travel to the relative safety of England. It took three weeks to complete the sea voyage.

They eventually arrived in Southampton. Mum had never been so seasick, and gave up most of her seafaring dreams after that.

They finally settled in London into the British lifestyle. Well, almost...they were learning how to adjust to the European way of life. Up until then they had worn mostly Indian clothes. It must have been a challenge for the parents, having six girls! Mum went to nursing school, graduated and eventually started working in a London hospital.

At the tender age of nineteen, she was young and beautiful with long black hair and attractive dark eyes. One of Mum's nurse friends had a brother and she introduced him to Mum. A dashing young Englishman, Tony, then 27 years of age, was handsome with turquoise blue eyes.

Mr. Carim had his own ideas about potential partners for his daughters. He forbade Fatima to see this Englishman any more. However, exposed to the freedoms taken so much for granted in the West, Mum had become an independent thinker. She decided, regardless of her father's wishes for her to be united to a fellow countryman of the family's choosing, that the Englishman was for her! He proposed after they courted secretly for a year, and they eloped. Mum had found her very own "Prince Charming"...or so it seemed at the time.

Her father was so outraged that he disowned his daughter, telling her never to see the family again. He was living in the West, but still within his own culture.

How odd that he fled the color prejudice of apartheid, and yet disowned his own daughter for falling in love with and marrying a white man.

The couple lived in London for two years, had their first child, Jasmine (Jas), then relocated away from the city to the seaside.

They moved to Torquay, two hundred miles from London, in the southwest of England - an area known as the "English Riviera." By this time Mum was known as "Tina" and had given up work as a nurse to become a full-time housewife. She and Tony began an interesting life, living to the rhythm of the Sixties' beat. They had two more children over the next two years: Lee (me) and then just a year later came the youngest, Mandy.

The son of a very traditional, wealthy English family, my father rebelled and was drawn to anything different and opposite to his very strict upbringing in stuffy boarding schools. His family owned one of the largest and most prestigious hotels in the North of England, some restaurants, a fishing fleet and various other business interests. In his day, children were expected to be seen and not heard. Consequently their lives were often void of simple love and affection. He once told Mum that the only hugs he got as a little boy were the times when the family's nanny put him on or took him off the potty. That lack of love and affection affected him for most of his life, and impelled him to take another course in life - one he hoped would fill the gaping void.

He experimented with, and often enjoyed, the temporary escape from reality that he found in smoking pot - or "Smokey Joes," as I renamed his "joints." These oversized cigarettes were rolled in profusion in our home. He kept his habit secret for quite a while, but eventually introduced his activity to Mum while in Torquay.

Over the years, Dad inherited a few small fortunes from his family, although he wasn't emotionally equipped properly to handle them or his young family responsibly.

We initially had a big house nestled at the end of a long lane with acres of woods behind. We had a nanny and a number of fine vehicles, including various sports cars. The nanny would address me as "Master Lee." Mum and Dad were very much part of the "in-crowd" then, of course.

It was about six years later when the funds dried up and reality finally set in. We moved to a different area and a small townhouse, in disrepair, on a busy main road. As the years went by Mum somehow juggled all that we didn't have, stretching every penny, and was able to make do. At times when our shoes were worn right through, she would cut cardboard and slip it in the shoes to cover the holes. I tried to avoid walking on gravel because it would hurt. Our clothes too often came from the charity shop. They may not have matched or fit properly, but at least we kept warm. To send us all into a deep sleep at night, she would sprinkle her magic sleeping dust over us. It always worked just like magic (If we opened our eyes or talked after she sprinkled us, the spell would be broken).

The fancy parties, luxury cars, and the nanny were all gone. Like most children we adjusted quickly. Tina & Tony acquired many friends of all ages and backgrounds whose hair, clothes styles and colors covered the whole spectrum. Our home at times was like a hippie festival gathering. Looking back, that's because it probably was one!

Mum would wear (just one of her often-colorful displays) a fancy purple-and-black-diamond- pattern, skin-tight cat suit, with black ballet slippers; Dad would sport brown work boots with purple trousers, an orange jumper, long hair and an earring, and that actually was to the PTA meetings! "Searching" was a word they often used. Others I used to hear bandied around were "groovy," "far-out, man!" "tripping," "cool," "heads!" "hippies!" "like...wow!" and my dad's favorite greeting: "Hey, nut!"

"Search" was what they did, as in... "the meaning of life!" After "Smokey Joes" came Transcendental Meditation, which all three of us children learned. Mum continued with TM. Dad enjoyed the more immediate gratification he got from his smoking, through which he escaped reality much of the time. It was about then that Mum realized she needed more from life for her children and herself. It was all fun and games while they were young, but at some point they had to grow up, even though Dad didn't want to...

Four years later, having listened to a sixteen-year-old guru from India, Mum received "knowledge"- that is, she was initiated as a devotee and had been taught specific meditation techniques. It was a significant and positive change for her. For the time, she truly found peace in her life and heart, independently from Dad. Shortly thereafter she announced we were all going to become vegetarians. At first it was largely tofu and aduki beans with brown rice and soy sauce. With time and experience, though, her many creations would make even an unenlightened heathen steak-eater opt to try her vegetarian dishes of delight.

Dad continued his search in life, relishing the advantages of adulthood but still not dealing well with the accompanying responsibilities.

The arguments increased, as did their frustrations with each other. I was fourteen when they finally decided to separate. He stepped out of our lives and met with us now and again over the years, though he initially only lived a mile away. He pursued his desire of building a boat and sailing off into the sunset. He then inherited a further small fortune, divorced Mum, abandoned building a boat and bought one instead. He eventually and literally sailed off to fulfill his personal dream, ending up in the Caribbean for a while. Mum always loved him and she never re-married.

I met up with him nine years later in 1993 in Brighton, England, at a pub. I was returning to England for a few weeks' vacation from the U.S. and arranged to meet him. It was a slightly awkward meeting. He was then sixty-four and his girlfriend looked to be in her early thirties. He had a huge, dangling earring on his left ear.

He ordered a pint of beer. I chose an orange juice. He took a moment and then said, "After all that you've seen and all that I have taught you, how can you have turned out to be so straight?" "I suppose I'm just a rebel!" I replied.

Mum was not afraid of hard work and did all she could to keep us clothed and fed. To augment the income during the summer months, she would pile the three of us into one room and rent out our bedrooms. Our house was now a "Bed-and-Breakfast." The morning air was filled with the scent of bacon and eggs and burning toast. The guests would always get first dibs on the only bathroom. During other summers, Mum would rent our rooms to foreign students, mostly seventeen to twenty years of age.

At these times I was put outside to sleep on a couch under the French glass panel cover, just outside the back kitchen door. I was woken up before the students so I could come in the house and get ready for the day, before they hogged the bathroom. I was about fifteen years old at the time and quite adaptable to the whole situation, as were we all. Mum would also teach English at the students' school during the summer. The students were always much more fun to have around than the Bed-and-Breakfast guests, who were usually a lot older. The students were more adaptable. Two male Italian students gave me pointers on clothes, dancing and style. I fell in love with the Swedish girls whenever they came to stay, although they clearly thought of me as just a nice English boy.

Mum was truly a Mum to many! She cooked amazing foods like Special "Beans-à-la-Mum" on toast. It was quite basic, but tasty. Heinz baked beans were added to frying onions, a little sugar, and a tiny pinch of chili for zest, cooked and served on buttered toast. It was wonderful! My school friends always craved this simple dish. She also cooked Malaysian cuisine and Indian curries for as many as fifty people in our house at a time. We sat on pillows around a tablecloth laid across the floor, and wherever else there was a place to squeeze into. It was a great time for building memories! These were not just meals for friends, they were events or "spreads!" Mum loved putting them on. The array of foods - colored rice, salads, chutneys, sauces, breads - made them veritable feasts.

The music ranged from Simon and Garfunkel, Cat Stevens, Pink Floyd and Joan Baez to Genesis, Santana, Led Zeppelin, classical, Jean Michelle Jarre, jazz and much more besides (I especially remember "Snow Flakes are Dancing" by Tomita and "Songs in the Key of Life" by Stevie Wonder, both of which we took with us to India). These events were quite exciting and peaceable. The drinks would flow, the conversation was lively and music filled the air. Some of my parents' friends must have traveled a lot, as I'd often hear them discussing their trips.

Friends on hard times always had a place to lay their weary heads, even if it was on the couch in the front room. With all there was to do, Mum still found time to give us love and hugs and make us laugh.

She was an extraordinary woman who lived an extraordinary life. She touched the lives and hearts of many people. She always had an ear to listen and a shoulder for her friends to cry on. She loved people and people loved her. Bristol was where she eventually settled and found her own space, peace, and quiet. She loved the rolling hills and the rich green countryside in that part of England.

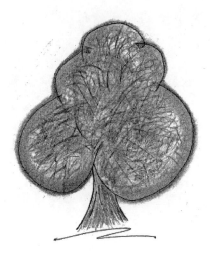

Chapter 2

I Get the Call

It is a usual sunny morning in Tampa, Florida, and I am up early as usual. I feel happy watching the sunbeams bathe the room with the golden warmth of the tropical sun. Breakfast is the usual quick event: a piece of toast and a swig of coffee, and then out of the door I go. "I owe, I owe, it's off to work I go!" I incant under my breath as I walk to my car. I get into the usual morning traffic and still wonder "why do Americans drive on the opposite side of the road?" I head west along Bearss Avenue. The palm trees displayed in people's yards stand high above the fences and walls, the drooping green palms looking perfect against the blue sky in the bright sunshine.

I make a quick stop in a drive-thru to get another coffee. The server is wide-awake and has no doubt been here since 05:00 a.m. She gives me an enthusiastic, "Have a nice day now!" as I leave the window and head back down the road towards the office.

Cars are everywhere on this bright morning. I continue on to a traffic light and quickly stomp the gas peddle, just managing to scoot through the intersection on the yellow light without spilling my coffee. In Tampa, when the light is green you go; when yellow, you go faster; when red, you go very fast.

The usual "good mornings" are exchanged twelve or so times as I walk into the pristine offices. Entering the spacious marble foyer, with its water fountain glistening under the fifty-foot high glass skylight, always leaves me with a good feeling.

One day I'll say, "Good snoring to you?" or something of the sort, just to see if anyone actually hears what I say, or indeed cares. Would they still automatically reply "Good morning," I wonder? I get situated, greet a few fellow employees, and am ready to start the day.

I am pleased about my recent promotion and my very own ground floor corner office with large plate glass windows overlooking the lush tropical greenery. It's a nice change from the little cubicle I used to share. My recent promotion meant a lot to me and I'm glad to be here now.

I'm all ready for the phones to start ringing and the fax paper to start flowing; for e-mails to start arriving and reports needing filing, and clients with whom to talk. The day normally goes by in a blur. But first I have to attend the usual morning meeting.

Suddenly my cellular phone bursts into life with a pleasant little tune, announcing my sister Jasmine from England. She blurts out something incomprehensible and I ask her to slow down. I can't understand a thing she is saying. Jas explains that Mum is going to have to undergo emergency brain surgery tomorrow, Thursday, because she has just had a stroke. The doctor is not sure about the outcome and has suggested that all family members should be present. He does not feel she is going to get through this very well, if at all.

My legs suddenly feel like lead weights. I sit down. "Lee, *please* get the first flight here. *Come home!*" Jasmine implores me. While listening to this mind-numbing news, I try to calm her down as she struggles to contain her emotions and then bursts out crying, I understand why she feels so overwhelmed.

16

My mind flashes back...

Only nine months ago I was in England for three weeks helping Mum get through her radiation treatment for lung cancer, which thankfully, went into complete remission. Not long before that I was there speaking at my younger sister Mandy's funeral.

Mandy had died suddenly due to a reaction to her medication. She and her husband had been at the hospital most of the night because she had severe stomach pains. She was administered some fairly strong pain medication given to her by the same hospital one time before for the same condition. She was very tired by the time they returned home early in the morning and slept into the afternoon. Her husband tried to wake her to have some lunch. She asked him to let her sleep for another hour. When he came back to wake her up, she had already passed away. That devastated all of us and broke Mum's heart.

Just four months before that, my father had died after losing a two-year battle with cancer. We'd only learned of his actual condition a few days before he died.

I tell Jas that I'll call with the flight details as soon as I have any. I try to console her in some fashion as my tears well up inside. I hold them back. "I'll be there as soon as I can, I promise!" After I hang up the phone, I try to comprehend all that this news means and what needs to be done next. I walk over and close my office door, sit back down, and cry my heart out.

I gather my thoughts and begin to pull myself together. I have to get into action. If the worst happens there will be much to sort out. If things go well, Mum may need help just to get organized at home. I think about getting time off, deciding to ask for three weeks of emergency family leave, thinking I might be back sooner. I'd have to wait and see.

I call a few close friends to relay the news. I leave a few messages, and feel comforted by words of support, concern and prayer. I've got to get a few administrative things in order and a back-up plan, in case the situation doesn't work out as well as I hope it will. My first move is to go and chat with my supervisor. There are no questions, and with care and concern he advises me to do whatever I need to do. Otherwise, they look forward to seeing me back here in three weeks. I return to my desk and log onto the internet to start searching for flights.

With only a day's notice, the flight costs are simply out of this world, even with the special rate for family emergencies. Worse, still, there are no outbound flights available for a week or more from Tampa. I may have to fly from Orlando (over an hour's drive away) or possibly even New York.

I get a call back from my friend, Dan. He is saddened by this news. I explain to him, among other things, my immediate flight dilemma. He happens to have a special flight membership with a major air carrier and says he will call back shortly. I hang up and my mind races with all I need to do. Contacting other friends to arrange transport to the airport gives me comfort since I am doing something positive and moving forward with a plan, even if it is sketchy at this point.

I'm done after ten minutes and, as I stare out of the window, I drift off thinking about brain surgery for Mum and contemplating my understanding of a stroke and the many possible implications of this new development. The thoughts are not pleasant ones. The phone rings. Dan has the flight details. Not only does he have flight details, he explains that he has thousands of extra air miles, and has gone ahead and used up a few of them for me with a return ticket to England.

Overwhelmed and in tears, I thank him for his kindness. I reflect that it's only when the chips are down that you truly find out who your real friends are.

The earliest flight available is Thursday in the late afternoon with a two-hour lay over in Atlanta and an arrival time in England at 06:30 a.m. GMT Friday morning. I thank Dan again and we arrange to meet at the airport first thing in the morning to get the ticket sorted. I call Jasmine back to give her the flight details. She is greatly relieved and says that she and her husband, Mike, will pick me up at the airport.

I think about the most important women in my life right now: my sister and Mum. They have never had the best relationship. They just don't seem to be able to get along.

I don't know why that is. Perhaps Dad not being around to give her that special sense of significance in the early years really affected Jas? Maybe she sought that from other people? Either way, she was always happier to do her own thing regardless of what Mum said. Thoughtful, soft and kind words were not always her gift.

Perhaps this situation will make the difference? I muse. They live relatively close by, certainly when seen from my perspective, and yet don't see each other very much. Their expectations of each other are not one and the same. How sad! Life is simply too short.

It all seems so silly and such a waste of time. But to those involved, the issues at stake are very important. I am aware of the fact that this is not easy for my sister, and I hope that at some point soon she will somehow reconcile her differences with Mum and see the same funny, wise, loving person I see. Then, I hope and pray, they'll be able to show tenderness to one another.

My thoughts drift on to consider the relationship that was between Mandy and Mum. There was often tension, particularly after Dad left, as things became more difficult. Obedience, or just being thoughtful and helping out, seemed to become a problem. It was as if Mandy, then thirteen, was depressed herself. We had a great friendship while we were growing up, and much fun as kids. If she had been sent to bed without dinner, I would make sandwiches, climb the ladder in the back of the house, tap on the window and hand over the goodies. Her little face would light up with a big smile.

Mandy loved horses most of all and always had a great time at riding school. Years later I wondered if that was because she received unconditional love from her animal friends.

She was very affected by our parents' separation, and it was at that time that she would often get into trouble. She had many arguments with Mum, had left home early and ended up marrying very young. For a while she, too, disowned fellow family members.

It took many years before she began to come around. Eventually, she and Mum began to communicate again and they gradually started to take advantage of the years they had now rather than dwelling on the ones lost. Perhaps that was why her sudden passing was so especially tragic for Mum?

~ ♦ ~

I call the front desk to forward all my office calls to a colleague then I sit in a sort of numbness, gathering my thoughts. I feel I will be useless at work and so, with a quick "goodbye," I rush out to the car. Somewhat distracted, I go straight home to organize and pack. It is a quick drive home and I don't hit anything.

My friend, Mike, who has just recently rented me a room in his house, arrives back from work. I explain to him and his girlfriend the situation, and that I will be back in two or three weeks. They are fine with whatever I need to do.

I throw a few of the warmest clothes into my suitcase. It has got to be cold in England in January. I put my address/contact books and some reading material into my carry-on bag.

I'm done in hardly any time.

It is a restless night and I have a million thoughts going on in my mind. I wake up early, shower and get ready to go... except the flight is not until the late afternoon. I have arranged to meet Dan at the airport to get the ticket sorted. With that taken care of so easily, I thank my friend. He says a tender prayer, and then rushes off to get to his office.

I drive back to my place, pack my things into the car, and decide to pay a last trip to a café bookstore to help pass the time. I order a steaming hot soy coffee latte, and go to the music section to see if there is something for Mum. She loves her music, and this keeps me occupied.

It is hard to believe that only a few months ago I was doing the same thing, getting coffee and picking out music, before I left for England to help her with the lung cancer decisions and treatment options.

Time passes so slowly today. I have a buddy, Joel, whom I have been picking up for work on some days. It occurs to me it'd be a good idea to just let him use the car while I'm away. This arrangement will work for both of us since he can then drop me off at the airport later. Before that, though, I also have to say goodbye to another good buddy, Ben. We chat, and he prays with me for strength, wisdom and courage. How blessed we are with true friends; they are gifts not to be taken for granted.

A childhood thought comes to mind out of nowhere…
(Flashback)
Mum often made us laugh. She has always been such a happy soul. From my youngest memories of childhood at age four or five, I remember her on the side of the bathtub bathing us. We would grab hold of her and pull her fully clothed into the bath with us. She would pretend to make the biggest fuss. We'd all laugh and laugh, and water would swoosh everywhere. She would do that at least once a week. What fun!

My head is a flood of thoughts and scenarios as I run them through my mind, trying to anticipate what to do first when I arrive. It definitely seems as though I have "ants in my pants" as I pace about, ready to go and meet Joel from work to drive me over to the airport. After the good-byes, the hugs and "we'll keep you in our prayers," the car and Joel disappear around the corner. I am on my own. Check-in and then up and away to Atlanta for two hours, and then an eight hour or so flight to England.

Chapter 3

The flight

I sit comfortably in my seat and buckle up. Just as I lean back I can see the next person struggling in the aisle five rows in front. What a huge carry on bag he has! Maybe he gets a special discount travel ticket if he has another family member in there? I wonder how that big bag could possibly fit in the overhead baggage compartment! With the expertise of a kind stewardess and another passenger, and a swift heave-and-jerk movement, the three of them lift and slide the bag and fill most of a compartment. None of the noise I expected comes from the bag. The stewardess acknowledges the assistance, and the helpful passenger smiles back weakly. He looks as though he may have just pulled a muscle. I wonder whether he'll be as keen to get it down? Bless his heart! But it was kind of him offer to help, I reflect.

I wonder for a moment how many on this flight are on business or on holiday; how many are traveling because of births, marriages or funerals or are perhaps going to see loved ones? Whatever the reason, we are all called to the skies on this day at this time. Mine is a mission to support and help my mum & sister. If I get asked the "where are you going to?" question, I'll just say to England to see family. I don't feel much like talking about it. I just want the next few hours to pass quickly, and hope that there aren't too many people on the Atlantic flight from Atlanta. I'm hoping I can stretch out a little over the (empty) seats next to me and sleep.

Such is the way things work out. I get aboard the second flight and lo and behold, I have all three seats to myself. Great! A reasonable chance of sleep is what this means to me.

The familiar push back in the seat happens as the plane lurches off the runway, heading for the sky in a hurry.

Mum's surgery is to be in the early evening on Thursday, possibly right now as we fly. I won't know until I get to the airport tomorrow whether she even made it through the operation. I close my eyes to pray. (He must be such a busy God, all around the world at this very moment. There are millions of people praying for millions of different needs, mercy, fear's, hurts, wants or desires twenty four hours a day, seven days a week, in hundreds of different languages and dialects all at the same time, day and night. How can he possibly hear mine? I hope my prayers are also worthy to be heard and acted upon.) Oh *please*, dear God, let my Mum come through this. Guide the doctors and nurses as they do their job. Please keep my sister strong and comfort her right now...and bring me to England safely please...A-men.

Perhaps, if I can't sleep, I'll watch an in-flight film to occupy my mind over the next few hours. I stare out into the emptiness of the blue sky. I am reminded of my first flight with Mum...

It was a fun flight as I recall and an adventurous trip. It was the time in my life where she became not just a mum that I loved dearly, but a good friend with whom I liked spending time. I begin to think about some of those great times with Mum.

We once took a six-month trip to India...

My sisters didn't want to go, and Dad was able to look after them while we were away. I was sixteen years old and had worked doing all kinds of jobs during the summer to save funds, Mum did too. She had suggested that I could do what I was initially planning, which was to buy a motorcycle to ride around with friends, or I could use the funds on "the trip of a lifetime" to India. India sounded exciting and adventurous, so I opted for the trip.

(Flashback)

Thinking about it now…I close my eyes, and it's as if we are right *there*… It is early December 1975 and, with bags and music packed, we say our goodbyes and leave for London. The anticipation once at London's Heathrow airport is incredible. It is exciting enough just to see so many planes and people from every nation, but an added spectacle soon presents itself. A whole group of bald people in orange attire dances around, banging little drums and cymbals. They hand out flowers as they come through the airport terminal, singing to one another and everyone else to hurry: "You'd better hurry, oh hurry, hurry; oh hurry, hurry!" They soon go, obviously on a tight schedule themselves.

After the preliminaries we step into the massive body of the 400 ton 747 Jumbo jet. It is our very first flight in a jet. We are in what seems like a huge corridor twenty feet wide with seats as far as the eye can see in both directions. We have seats next to a window. Mum asks me how this thing can possibly get off the ground. I assure her with apparent conviction that I've seen one take off… on television once. Reassured by my confident explanation, she nods nervously, squeezing my hand. I ask her to sit back and loosen her grip. I talk her into holding on to the armrest for a moment.

I am excited, as any young man would be. It takes about an hour before all are on board, seated and ready. The stewardesses do their survival review and procedures. Mum starts looking for exit doors and a survival vest to put on; I calm her down. As the stewardesses also prepare to sit and the plane begins to move away from the terminal, it seems as though Mum is going to cry. She asks, "Are we flying now?"

The Jumbo maneuvers to the end of the runway. The four huge Rolls Royce engines release their tremendous energy as the crew holds the brakes for a static start and increase the power to the point that the engines are screaming. It is at about this point that Mum wants to go to the bathroom. "Not now, Mum," I insist, "We have to take off first!" Her eyes are as wide as plates. Suddenly the brakes are released and the huge jet surges forward, anxious to get going. The runway moves by faster and faster until we reach about 180 mph. As the engines roar and the nose lifts, Mum grips my arm so tight it hurts. We sink back into our seats as this amazing ship of the sky lifts off the ground, defying gravity once again: Eastbound...we are going to India! The wheels clunk as the undercarriage folds away. Mum's response at this time with a big grin on her face is, "Wow, far out! We're flying! Isn't it amazing?"

Twelve hours later, we touch down in India, excited and tired. We get through the airport hustle and bustle and pick up our bags from luggage reclaim.

The main airport doors open. The sights, sounds, the crowds of people, smells, heat and volume of noise is all just incredible!

Mum stands in disbelief, taking in the mesmerizing view outside the airport. It is still hot and dry at about 4:00 p.m. We look around to get our bearings, trying to spot a taxi stand. All of a sudden, we find ourselves to be in the centre of quite a commotion, and are almost knocked over by a crowd of young and old skinny men. They have odd matching clothes: what looks like a tablecloth for trousers or wrap and a curious little cloth, wrapped around itself to form a sort of circular rope, placed on top of their heads. They all want to carry our cases! We wave for a taxi, and the entire crowd starts shouting and waving too, as if it were now their idea, sticking their hands out for a tip as the black and yellow taxi pulls up. The driver jumps out and starts shouting at the men, who voice a few words back and then, as quickly as they appeared, all turn and run, bumping into and tripping over themselves and each other to get back to the exit doors.

"Velcum to Dehli," says the proud cab driver (in a thick Indian accent), smiling and wobbling his head sideways as he speaks. "Frum vhere arrrre yu cuming, actually?" he asks, chucking the bags into the boot and the front of the car. "England!" Mum replies, all bubbly.

She was about ten years old the last time she was here. We get into the car, an old British Ambassador. There are no AC controls and no seat belts, but it does have a steering wheel! Mum gives the taxi driver the address for the Royal Hotel, and he gets moving excitedly.

He turns on the music. Say what? Sounds just like Indian restaurant music. Shame there is no food in the car! We hurtle down the street on the left, and then dodge an overturned car in the street. Our happy driver beeps his horn at the unfortunate car for good measure! We are literally swerving around pedestrians and bicycles, cow's and what was that funny looking thing that just went by? A three-wheeled scooter? No, a rickshaw!

All the cars on the road are swerving around something. Everyone is part of the same organized and utter chaos they call "traffic" here, screaming and beeping their horns and waving their fists. I reflect that, to start driving a taxi here, you must just have to be brave enough to show up at the office, then they give you keys and off you go! I'm sure you don't even need a driver's license.

I wish our driver wouldn't keep looking back as he talks and drives in this mess! Mum says she thinks she's got one of her headaches coming and starts laughing and covering her eyes.

We drive through what looks like the rough end of town as we avoid another cow walking in the road. The buildings are old and dilapidated and almost on top of one another. "The sun peels the paint off," says Mum. The street is crowded with people going in all directions. Some are shouting from shops, while others are offering their wares from bicycle baskets. Mum starts to explain that she recalls such places as a kid. People tried to avoid this area of town at night because of the danger. I notice that it is dry and quite dusty. Suddenly, the taxi stops. Mum signals quietly to roll up the windows. (This will apparently protect us from robbers and other terrible dangers.) Just then the driver says, with a smile and a head wobble, "Vell, here ve are! ...Ve are at the Rrrroyal Otel!...

Arrr u readi to goh?" Mum starts looking for the address. Go? Here? Obviously the driver has made a mistake! She shakes her head ... no, apparently not! This *is* it!

Mum has a bewildered look on her face. She hadn't seen a brochure, but assumed that the Royal Hotel in Delhi would be, ummm, well... more - "Royal," I suppose. We give the driver a few extra rupees, "Oh, I'm thanking you sooo very much! May your moments of time here be blessed!" he enthuses with a head wobble. He leaves and we stand there gazing at the Royal Hotel, which evidently is distinguished by virtue of its name alone. Mum announces that she really does have one of her headaches coming. She mumbles in disbelief as we start moving towards the scruffy main entrance. It is only then that we notice one of the main front doors is partially hanging off.

As I struggle with the cases, Mum goes on ahead to check into the room, nearly exhausted by this time. I arrive with all the luggage and place it on the... errr...sandy floor. I look around the square reception area where I notice that the walls are bare and the dirty yellow colored paper is peeling off on the inside. This place hasn't seen paint in over twenty years! The small wooden desk, by which Mum is standing while engaged in conversation, is almost antique in its worn unpolished state. The wood is splitting and discolored on the sides from hands holding on to it. I imagine that guests over the years needed to hold themselves steady once the clerk announced they were actually going to be charged for staying here.

I pick up the conversation at the point at which Mum is explaining to the manager, who apparently has also been on the same spot for a considerable length of time, that we did not, in fact, bring him any duty-free whisky from the airport. The manager now adopts the familiar head wobble, too. They only have one room left on the fourth floor, which is a "suite" (this'll be interesting...) with a view of the main street. The reception looks like a film set. A very old one.

The manager points toward the stairs and then points up. There is no elevator. Well, we can manage a night or two, long enough to get over the jetlag and to get a little more acclimated. Mum walks ahead of me, mentioning a hot shower and some sleep. We climb up the stairs, looking for the number twelve. There is a waist-high wall on the left and one can clearly see some of the city from here, although it is slowly getting dark now. I struggle breathlessly to the top of the stairs at which point I hear Mum-speaking French! Number twelve has a padlock on it and, as she opens the lock and the door, I see something with little legs scurry across the dusty concrete floor. I don't say anything to Mum. The windows are wide open. Mum snorts.

"They must be joking!" she exclaims. We look throughout the "suite." It is predictably basic, with the shower area consisting of one pipe coming out of the wall and no showerhead. There is one sheet on each bed, and a lowly light bulb dangling brightly from the ceiling. Mum goes out and down the stairs to see the manager but returns about fifteen minutes later.

There are no refunds, and it is such a hassle to go find another place at this point. "Let's just make do. I'm exhausted," she announces. We do our best to settle down. Mum goes in to take her hard-earned steaming hot shower, then a scream emanates from the bathroom: "THERE IS NO HOT WATER!" she shrieks. I suggest this hotel should be considered to be like an...err...a camping trip, perhaps? But this doesn't do much to change her frame of mind.

The area comes to life when we turn out the lights a short while later. It is a long night occupied with swatting mosquitoes, the general noise of people laughing and shouting, new smells of burning charcoal, incense, curry and car fumes and the cars, motorcycles and rickshaws beeping their horns at anything on the road, including the cows. Now then, where did that hairy little thing go that scurried across the floor earlier, I wonder?

We awake to a hot sunny new day, refreshed. Looking at the room from a different perspective in the daylight, it doesn't look as bad in the daylight...actually, it looks much worse! We might change to something better before tonight if possible. Right now, though, we are excited to start the day. Almost breakfast time! "What's for breakfast in India?" I wonder. I'm dressed, with my sandals on, in no time. Mum is taking a little longer. I offer to venture outside the bedroom door as I hear some English voices in the corridor.

It is a bright and noisy day. The voices turn out to belong to two teachers on holiday from Cornwall in the south of England. What a small world! Jack & Gary have been in the Royal Hotel for a week already. They talk about the area, and they have no concerns at all. "The people are quite friendly, there's lots to do and there are good places to eat locally, but do be careful of the water," they warn me, "Just don't drink it!" says Gary. At this point Mum comes out and introduces herself. They say they will accompany us to the hotel entrance and point us to an area where they know there are places to eat. As we get to the end of the corridor I say I need "to go" before we depart. Jack points the way to a bathroom just down two steps to the left. I walk off quickly.

I can see the traffic as I look over the wall to my right. I peer inside a couple of doors and see nothing, although I think it is pretty nice to have foot washes in one of the rooms. I've never seen that before - neat little sunken foot washing troughs all level to the floor. I try one out since my feet are already dirty from our dusty room floor.

Putting both feet into the narrow trough I pull the cord to release the water, which washes over them. I notice there are a number of troughs, six in a row - not surprising really, I ponder, when you consider how dirty it is everywhere. Perhaps lots of people come in here? We'll all probably have to stop in after we get back later today...

I hurry back, run into our room, and shortly after rejoin the assembled company. The others stop chatting as I return and announce that it must be breakfast time and, "oh, by the way, there isn't a bathroom room down there!" We slowly make our way downstairs. Jack points to the bathroom as we go past. I correct him politely: "no, that's the foot washing room, and I've just been washing my feet. It is a good idea!"

Howls of laughter ensue as the others explain that, in India, they use "squatty potties!" "You've just washed your feet in their toilet!" they guffaw. Evidently this is all quite humorous, judging by their inability to speak for the next couple of minutes, and the way they hold their stomachs and wahaaaa-haaa. After they recover from the laughter, Jack & Gary point out a few directions in which we might want to explore. They leave and we go our way to find breakfast! (They're still chuckling as they walk away!)

"Lassi!" says Mum. I'm looking for a collie dog I remember from childhood TV, as Mum points to a tiny little stall where there are huge red pots filled with a white, milky substance. Little clay cups are stacked invitingly to the left and right of these. "I remember this!" she says excitedly. "There is sweet lassi and salt lassi. It is goats' milk yogurt with sugar or with salt." I opt to try the sweet one. It is really good, so I have another (you can do this with everything there, if you feel so inclined, as it is all so cheap by our standards). After drinking the contents, you throw the cup to the ground. It is made of unfired clay and will eventually melt back into the ground, I'm told. Mum is down memory lane, savoring the taste not of today, but of years ago. She is happy, fondly remembering a time I will never know or see. It is good to see her so excited.

We spend another night at the "Royal" and the following afternoon we head off to the train station. We are taking a three-day train trip through India down to Madras in the far south. Mum has booked bunk beds, too! An old friend of Mum's, Sherrie, is on an Indian dance course down there. She is being sponsored by the British government, and will spend one year learning so that she can teach classes of the same when she returns to England. We will stop by and see her. We depart from the hotel. Perhaps someone else will find the thing scurrying around the room? When it grows bigger and hairier, perhaps...who knows?

It is another manic drive to the trains and complete mayhem in the station. I have never seen anything like it. Mum gives me instructions, which are: to hold on to one another and the bags. The noise of the general crowd is loud, almost deafening, but it is

35

exciting to see so much happening. The bag carriers don't have carts but they have their heads, with those circle cloths on to soften the load. Mum points out a man. This quite skinny fellow coils a scarf onto his head and then lifts a huge trunk, bigger and heavier than he is himself, and balances it on his head. Wow! Amazing! I'm very happy for him! I'll just pull ours along on its wheels, if that's okay.

Eventually we find our train. It's huge, and the main engine is a large impressive-looking shunter diesel engine. The well-dressed guard helps us find the correct carriage.

He sits us in our single-slatted wooden chairs opposite one another, next to the window overlooking the platform. People are brushing right past us in the aisle. There are two four-seater benches opposite facing each other. An Indian family is sitting there, looking and smiling at us. I see that Mum is a little worried and I ask the train guard about the private cabin with our bunk beds. He says, "Oh, just lifting yourr veeet, please, and zslide up the vwood to the middle peece. It vwill lock into place, and then doing the same ubuve your heads, pleeze, vhen nite time is cuming, also. So, thank yuu." He starts to walk off. Mum asks him to wait! Where is the mattress, the blankets, the private cabin? He looks at the tickets again, saying, "No, no, youu are quvite correctt. This is it. This is your sleeping right here, isn't it! No blankets, no mattress. Thank yuu berry much!" his head wobbling as he walks off into the general chaos of bags and a sea of people. "This promises to be an interesting trip!" Mum declares, as she stares at the tickets in disbelief.

Our window is open and there are five horizontal bars stretching from left to right. The street salespeople are in prime time and selling their food and wares through the bars. It all looks nice and smells wonderful, but Mum shakes her head, "best not to chance it!" Suddenly we hear the interesting sound of a man coming down the aisle towards us shouting what sounds like, "Coppy, coppy, cheye walla! Coppy, coppy, cheye walla!" He is holding a cylindrical container with a little tap on the side and a long chain attached to the container at one end to a little tin cup on the other.

The family to our right stops him and hands over some change as he fills up the little cup with steaming hot tea or "chai." He is still shouting his favorite words and the drinker has no time to relax and enjoy the beverage. You have to drink up and let him move on. He quickly wipes the cup and offers it to the next person, Mum. Mum smiles at him and wishes him well.

Sleeping is "fun," and Mum makes a number of creative comments about it over the next three days. I sleep on the top bunk. We take clothes out of our suitcase to soften the bench and to lay over us at night. We work it out so that I stay awake at night to watch that no one steals from our bags while Mum keeps watch during the daytime as I sleep.

We get to know the family opposite us, who kindly share their many home cooked meals with us. As people from the West, we stand out, and people for the most part are very helpful and eager to make our acquaintance. Mum is having a ball, and by the end of the train trip she too starts doing... the head wobble. It is an interesting time for us, mother and son. We have never spent this much time together in a foreign environment, and I begin to see

her in a new light: she's such an entertaining traveling companion!
A sort of automatic protective sixth sense goes on inside me as
well. Out here, each of us is all the other has...

"Madras," declares the sign. We have arrived! Within an hour
of being here we check in to a YMCA. It is clean, air-conditioned
and has real beds, hot showers and no squatty (foot washing)
potties. We are the only guests here. We lie down for a quick rest
and fall into a deep asleep.

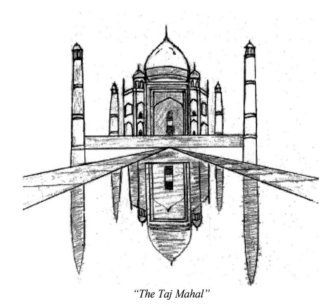

"The Taj Mahal"

Chapter 4

Back in England

The captain announces our final approach to Gatwick Airport. He then gives the weather advisory for England at this time. By the look of the solid blanket of gray clouds below, I already sense the need for rubber boots, an umbrella and maybe a boat. In any case, it is certainly wonderful weather for ducks!

I get through the short line and show my British passport to the customs lady. I grab my other bag from baggage reclaim and head over to the green light and on to the exit. Is Mum still alive? As my mind *snaps* back into the present reality, I begin to focus now on whatever task lies ahead, to be strong for my sister and Mum. I spot my sister and her husband. We all hug and Jas begins to cry. I don't want to think the worst. I try to read her eyes to shed some light, they reveal nothing. "How is Mum?" I ask immediately. "She made it through the surgery and is in intensive care right now," she replies.

It has been a tiring couple of days for Jasmine and Mike and a very early start for them today, to drive nearly one hundred and seventy miles to be here by 06:30 a.m. We make our way to the parking lot and begin a three-hour journey to Bristol and directly to the head trauma unit at Frenchay Hospital.

As we pull out onto the road and then on to the M25, the sky is dark gray and the rain is pouring. It is a typical cold, dreary English January day. Now, I know why I live in Florida. This only confirms it!

My sister gives me the rundown of events, to the best of her knowledge, leading up to Mum's current situation and the last couple of days. From what she understands, Mum had apparently not been feeling so good and had been to see her doctor, who promptly sent her to the BRI hospital for overnight observation. Mum called to advise my sister and expected all would be well by the following day.

In the morning, when the nurses came to give her breakfast, they noticed that Mum couldn't reply. She just stared at them and then suddenly fell sideways unconscious in the bed. Realizing something drastic was happening, the nurses quickly examined her and concluded, in the light of the symptoms, that she had possibly had a stroke. They contacted a doctor and rushed her to the X-ray room and took a brain scan. The doctor saw a dark mass in her head. Fearing that a burst or blocked blood vessel could do even more damage, a brain operation was deemed the best option. It needed to be done, and done soon. She would have to be transferred from the BRI to Frenchay hospital, on the other side of the city, which is where brain surgery takes place. The hospital contacted my sister at this point and explained the gravity of the situation, and what they were going to do. Jasmine contacted me as quickly as she could. She called her husband and they both left work and drove the sixty miles to Bristol to be with Mum.

We continue driving and chatting, trying not to reflect on the reasons that I was here before so recently. We catch up with some small talk, and soon give up on that since we are all pretty tired. Jasmine puts her head down, curls up in the back seat and slips into a deep sleep. I talk to her husband to make sure he stays awake and alert. It is a tough three hours' drive with rain pouring down all the way. We eventually exit the M25 joining onto the M4 and then finally the M23, Bristol is not far away now.

I recognize some of the landmarks as we approach Bristol. We follow some of the smaller city roads, which lead us directly to Frenchay Hospital. A big blue hospital sign points towards Frenchay as we finally arrive. Mike parks the car and we run through the rain to the main doors. It looks like an old-fashioned school complex, with red brick Second World War barracks. It is a single storey building with very long corridors interconnecting other buildings and wards. We head to a ward at the very end of what must be the longest corridor I have ever seen, seeming to be at least three quarters of a mile long. We pass other visitors, doctors, and an emergency team wheeling a patient somewhere. I struggle for a moment with tears welling up inside as we approach the intensive care ward. We push through the swinging doors and walk into a fairly narrow entrance, which then widens to beds on both left and right, almost like a dormitory. Drip bags, electronic boxes, and sad faces greet us. Directly ahead of us, at the other end of the room, is a small group of five beds. It's the critical care area, and there's Mum. Bless her! She looks sound asleep.

I stand at her bedside. It is a shock to see such a large incision on the right side of her head, her scalp held together with what look like big staples. The hair on that same side has nearly all been shaved. There are various machines, pumps, and drip bags on stands, and most of them are in some way plugged into or attached to her. Now and again one of the systems makes a high pitched beeping sound, out of tune with all the other beeping systems I now notice around the ward. A nurse comes over and introduces herself. She explains the stage Mum is at in the process of post brain surgery.

Mum came out of surgery last night and initially responded after a few hours, but was in a delirious state of mind. She since has fallen back into a deep sleep, which is really not a sleep, but the effects of the anesthetic. If she does not respond after today, under the circumstances it may be an indication of serious brain damage.

The nurse invites us to come and ask her any questions. She answers us, points to the waiting room and the café, and then leaves us with Mum and the incessant beeping. Jas holds Mike tight and cries, feeling sad, tired and powerless to do anything. We gather three chairs and sit by the bed. As I look around at patients in this ward, there are others also gathered around their loved ones who are in similar or maybe even worse predicaments.

I stand, hold and stroke Mum's hand, and just start to talk to her in a normal tone of voice. First, I tell her who I am and that I am here from sunny Florida. I explain that she needs to wake up and that it is important for her to do so. I tell her how much she is cared about and loved. I suggest that she squeeze my hand if she can hear. Nothing! I continue talking in soft tones regardless, stroking and gently but confidently squeezing her hand [I silently hope and pray that this is not "it" for Mum; that she is not in some way locked in a twilight zone, able to hear and not respond].

We decide after an hour to go for some refreshments since we are now all pretty tired. We chat over tea and biscuits about the immediate game plan. Mike and Jas will return to work tomorrow now that I am here.

I will call and update them as the days go by and they will come at weekends and whenever possible. Later this afternoon they will need to drive my bags and me back to Mum's place. I will then return to Frenchay by bus first thing in the morning.

As we walk back to Mum's ward, I realize that our situation is just one of many and to each family here, of which there are many, their particular concern is the most important concern in the world to them.

We arrive back at Mum's bedside and take up our same positions. I continue to hold her hand and talk. A nurse comes over in the meantime, and quite firmly goes through her routine of talking and asking questions to Mum. She loudly announces who is present: "Your son is here from America!" She states emphatically. She continues with other encouraging words and then proceeds to ask her what day it is, who the Prime Minister is; where is Mum and why is she here? Even I have to think about the answer to some of the questions for a moment.

Mum stirs. The nurse encourages us to just keep talking after she leaves and assures us she will return in a little while. We do as instructed. A short time later, we quickly motion the nurse to come over. Jas stands up and comes closer. Recognizing us during a few moments of consciousness, Mum smiles and cries at the same time. I squeeze her hand. We are here by her side, just as she was by ours many times as children. Indeed, as she would be now if the roles were reversed.

She drifts back into a sleep. We wipe our tears and continue to encourage her until late. The nurses feel positive about her awakening, and suggest we come back first thing in the morning. That is all Mum can do for the moment. We kiss her forehead, and leave her in good hands.

Jas and Mike drop me off at Mum's apartment. We hug our goodbyes, and they continue on the sixty or so miles to get home. Bless them! This is not the time to discuss all eventualities with Jas. At some point I know we need to, but timing is everything. It seems surreal walking back into this home, having been here so recently - or so it feels. The scent of Mum's cooking lingers in the air, just enough to know it smells like Mum's. The place is clean and organized, as usual.

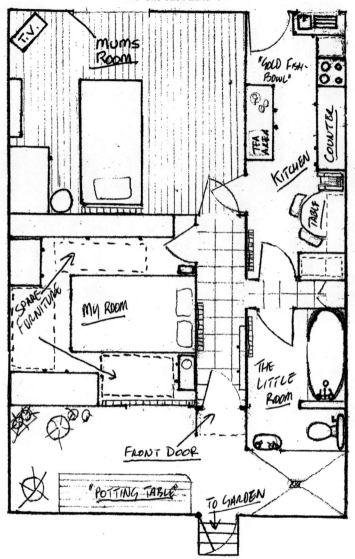

"The lay out of Mum's home"

45

Chapter 5

Back at Mum's Place

I put my bags and things in the bedroom and, with my priorities in order, I put on the kettle for a nice cup of tea. I know where everything is and the milk is good, too. It seems unreal to be here right now at this time, but here I am. I decide to call a couple of friends quickly, to let them know what is going on. Florida is five hours behind the U.K.

Mum has a nice one-bedroom garden flat that is fairly simple. It has a long entrance hall which leads from the front door to the lounge area. First right is a short hallway, with a kitchen door on its left and the bathroom to its right. Backing up the corridor again, Mum's bedroom (currently mine) is on the left. A king-sized bed fills up most of the space. The window overlooks her proud garden.

Entering the large sitting room from the hall, the tall sash window straight ahead overlooks the back lane. Lace curtains hang down from ceiling to floor and there are window shutters that can be closed from the inside, making the room almost dark during the day. To the left is an attractive fireplace and, turning right, a second entrance leads into the long, narrow kitchen.

In the kitchen a door with a frosted pane of glass opens from here onto the narrow back lane and this, together with the big, clear window above the sink, lets a lot of light into the room. Bouncing off the yellow walls, daylight lends this room a particularly cheerful atmosphere. Plants grace the windowsill.

I have no idea at this point how much time I am going to spend in this flat during the coming months, more specifically in this kitchen or - "the goldfish bowl," as it became known between friends. (From the back lane, through the large window, one neighbor remarked that I could always be seen there, very often sitting at Mum's round pine table at the far end of the room. For months on end my world shrank pretty much to encompass simply the space between these four walls.)

I sit in the lounge on the big white couch opposite the fireplace, with the window on my right. An old trunk serves as a coffee table. I switch on the TV to see the English news. I recognize some of the newscasters from years gone by. They are just older. Nothing is of particular interest and it is certainly not inspiring. I turn it off and think of who I need to call for Mum. I go on a hunt for her address books and start to get things organized and planned for the morning. As I prepare for bed, it's cold, so I leave my socks on and hop in to bed. I have had so many thoughts that I've just about worn myself out. Tiredness comes over me, like a sprinkle of magic sleeping dust, and I drift off as my mind finally disengages from the brain.

I get an early start, and head out of the front door. To go to town and look for the right bus to get to Frenchay Hospital, I have to go down the very steep St. Michael's Hill. From this vantage point, standing at the top, one can see over the city of Bristol and out to the green countryside in the far distance. But I won't linger for long since it is raining.

I walk through the modern busy city center. Quickly locating the correct bus stop, I am soon off to Frenchay. It is a twenty-minute ride. As we whiz through, I realize I have forgotten how narrow some of the streets are when cars are parked on either side of the road. Often there is only enough room for one car, even though it is a two-way street. We stop a few times to drop off and pick up passengers. I am dropped off at the bus stop just outside the hospital grounds. It's not too difficult to find an entrance door and the main corridors leading to the three-quarters-of-a-mile-long sloping corridor to Mum's ward.

I slowly push the swinging doors open and enter, hoping and praying that Mum is doing better today. Oh, I hope she is! It is busy here first thing in the morning with the nurses' shift change. The night nurses are updating the day nurses on each patient's condition and preparing for the doctors' walk-around. There's Mum in her same area. I kiss her forehead and squeeze her hand. She squeezes back, awake and all smiles, tears filling her eyes as she thanks me for coming. I let her know that it's okay and that I'm glad that I can be here.

I am holding back my own tears and I have to take a deep breath. "How are you feeling?" I ask her, "Did you sleep well?"

"Yes," she replies, "I did. It's busy here at night. Have you had any breakfast yet? You must have some breakfast, Lee!" "I'll be fine, Mum," I reply, but I think "it is you we need to be thinking about!" "Is Jas coming back?" Mum inquires. "Yes, Jas assures me that she will be back in a few days, but she and Mike have to get back to work for the moment," I reassure her.

Mum's little hand is firmly gripping mine and her thumb is slowly moving side to side, rubbing my hand. She is feeling reassured, as we do when we are children and are held and comforted by our mothers. She then falls back to sleep.

A nurse comes over to introduce herself. She is pleasant, slim, and smartly dressed. All the nurses here wear little white paper hats that are hair-pinned on. She also wears a light blue knee-length cotton dress, gathered in the middle, with black stockings. A little silver watch hangs from her top left pocket, which holds a pen. With a smile she explains how Mum is getting on and that she has had a restful night. She reminds me of Mary Poppins! "This condition will need a few more days of monitoring before we know how she really is. We have heard you came from America to be here! That's jolly good of you to come all this way," she says with a warm smile. Then she turns and goes about her duties. Where is that spoonful of sugar??

I'm tired and still in a time warp. It is now 06:00 a.m. in the States. I decide it is indeed time for breakfast and a nice hot cup of tea. The café is up the long corridor past the waiting room on the left. A number of other wards are on the right as I head out of the building, cross the road in the rain and enter the glass-enclosed area opposite. The café is large, roomy and busy. I arrive just as the staff are switching from serving breakfast to making lunch preparations. I manage to get the last scrapings of scrambled eggs and a piece of toast with strawberry jam, along with a nice cup of tea. I am surprised that everything is individually charged, including the little jam package, butter packs, ketchup and other condiments. I wonder whether I am going to be charged for napkins because they seem to ration them over here. Well, you can get one if you ask nicely or plead. Otherwise, I suppose you just use your sleeve. In the States you are welcome to any condiments at no additional charge and unlimited FREE refills of hot coffee, tea and sodas and napkins by the handful. It is at this moment I begin to realize how American I have become in my expectations. (I'll do my best not to say, "Ya'll have a nice day now, ya hear...!")

I carry my tray off to a table and sit alone wondering about so many things... who, what, why, where and how? I will call Mum's friends tonight and let them know when it would be good for them to visit. Right now isn't the best time, but perhaps as the nurse said it will be better in a few days time when she is clearer and more awake.

Hmmm... the tea is nice and hot. In America you're lucky if it's lukewarm, and no one's heard of the idea of adding milk to it, apparently. I look outside into the rain. It's coming harder now, streaming down the café window. It is strange to imagine that just the other day I was in the sun, surrounded by palm trees.

Mum loved coming to Florida. She used to come over for a month or two every Christmas, and she would look forward to the trip all year. She enjoyed the Disney places, but Sea World was her favorite theme park. One year she didn't feel so good and so I pushed her everywhere in a wheelchair. They have a disabled policy, meaning one can go to the front of any line to see shows and attractions, so it worked out quite well. Looking outside, I know why she loved coming over. I'm so glad the opportunity was there while she was able to take advantage of it.

Upon my return to the ward, I find the nurses are trying to talk to Mum again. One explains there is a waiting room next door with comfy chairs to rest in. "Your mum is sleeping, so why don't you rest a bit," suggests Mary Poppins. I head to the empty waiting room, settle down and pick up a magazine to read, but quickly drift off into a deep sleep. A couple of hours later a nurse's assistant wakes me with a cup of tea and biscuits. How wonderfully British! There are a couple of other people sitting, too. I have no idea how long they have been here. I wonder whether I was sleep talking, drooling, or snoring... I don't know, and they probably won't tell. They're still here so it can't have been that bad, unless I've scared all but these two people away!

One lady asks if anyone would mind her turning on the television. There is some update coming on about a popular English TV soap opera. I'm not much of a TV addict, but I'm happy for her to put her show on. Conversation from that point is minimal as the TV takes over. Perhaps they are just trying to forget about what I did while I was sleeping?

I walk over to Mum's bed. She speaks a little more, but has no recollection of this morning. How curious this seems but apparently this sort of thing is quite normal, according to a nurse. I sit by Mum's side and talk to her throughout the day, taking a few tea breaks in between.

Over the next four days, nurses speak to Mum every time they come to her bedside to make adjustments, asking the same basic questions about the day, time, Prime Minister, and whether she knows where she is and why she is here. They do this to be sure that the patient, having had major brain surgery, is responding or thinking properly and making progress each day. It is important that Mum does not become delirious or unresponsive. If she does not respond well, they will take that as a probable complication. Thankfully, she starts to respond quite well, without too much difficulty, and continues to improve further.

After one particular chat with her, she almost convinces me that her ward is unconventionally busy after lights out. She explains that the nurses have a party every night, with flashing green disco lights, along with a night filming crew and their bright lights. She also "sees" patients walking about swapping and moving beds around! Over the next few days I have a couple of strange conversations with her. I'm not sure whether I should laugh or call a nurse for help! The constant questioning goes on.

It's quite subtle when she makes the transition from that peculiar state to a stable state of mind.

After a week and a half it is good to hear Mum laugh again. When I tell her about some of her thoughts and the green lights she thinks it is the funniest notion, and can hardly believe she has said those things. She explains that she was telling a nurse about a person who was moving from bed to bed, and the nurse removed the equipment that Mum thought was a person. Mum says, "Boy! These pills must do something funny to my head!"

After another week, she is recovering well enough to be moved to a non-acute care area, where they'll also now monitor her less active left side. It is likely that she will need physical therapy at the next hospital to get the full use of her left side again. I feel sure I will be here just a couple more weeks or so, to help her recover, and then I will return to the U.S.

I arrive early the next morning, have breakfast with a nice hot cup of tea and get to Mum just as she is finishing hers. She says, "I feel much better today, and my headache isn't as prominent as long as my left side improves." She reaches over, using her right hand to reposition her left hand over her stomach.

Mum's doctor walks over to us to talk to us. We are eager to hear what he has to say about the stroke and how soon she can recover and go home. He briefly introduces himself, speaking softly but confidently, and then says, "During the operation we discovered what happened to you was not the result of a stroke, but of the expansion of a brain tumor. It is malignant and it is beyond anything we can do. It is inoperable. I'm very sorry to have to tell you this... you have terminal brain cancer." [Silence!]

He is clearly disturbed to give us such news. With no further explanation, he advises me to call him in the morning. Then he hands me his card. I give a sort of knowing nod and, without another word, he backs up with his head lowered, turns, and quietly walks away.

SHOCK! I can hardly believe the words he just said. My mind goes completely blank for a few moments. I want to wake up from this horrible dream! My heart wants to scream out, "Nooooooo!! NOT MY MUM!" But this is for real! How alone this moment feels!

I reach for Mum's hand. She is still staring at the empty spot where the doctor just stood. We both start to come to our senses, tears welling up in our eyes. We cry and hug. It is okay. It is okay to cry out. We don't speak for a while: I sit back on the chair by the bed and hold her hand. Mum lies there, silent in distant thought.

I turn on my brave face and pray. I pray for a deep strength from within to get us through this time and whatever may lie ahead. I pray for courage most of all. It is not me lying there; it is my Mum. I have to be strong for her. Life will be different from this day forward. At the moment, I am unable to imagine just how different...

We sit quietly as the day passes uneventfully. Mum is quiet, more thoughtful than depressed, just trying more than anything to accept the news internally. I let her rest alone, while I leave to use a phone for a few minutes.

It is now my job to tell my sister. It is the toughest phone call I have ever had to make and this is going to be difficult. Her cell phone rings. "Jas, it's Lee," I begin. "Hey, Lee, how's Mum?" she enquires. As I begin to explain what the doctor has said, I can hardly get the words out myself. After a few moments Jasmine cries out, "No! NO!"

We can barely understand each other, both crying and talking at the same time. Finally she says, "You and I... are all that's left now. We only have each other Lee." "I'm here, Jas," I reply, "Don't worry. I'm here. Jas, call Mike will you?" "Yes, I will," she assures me, "We'll drive over later as soon as I can get hold of him. 'bye"...Click. I pull myself together, and walk back.

I sit by Mum, stroking her forehead for quite a while as she drifts off to sleep. She wakes later at about 6:00 p.m. She wants to know whether I'm okay. I say, "As much as you would expect one to be. More importantly, how are you?" "You know," she replies, "I'm okay for now. Of course I would rather not be in these circumstances, but I am. Lee, I have had a good run for my money. It has been a wild ride!"

Jasmine comes in and approaches Mum's bed, all puffy-eyed and crying. They hug as Mum strokes her head and softly assures her that she is feeling okay. It takes a little while for Jas to let go, but there is no hurry. Mike, too, hugs Mum and is similarly overwhelmed. We three sit, consoling one another and Mum, yet Mum seems more upbeat than any of us. The nurses are fully aware of the diagnosis and are tender around us at this moment. We can't just sit here all night, so I sound the tea alert! I walk off with Mike to the café before it closes for the night. I tell him that I will call and chat with the doctor in the morning and let him and Jas know the bottom line.

Later, we kiss Mum goodnight, telling her we love her. Then Jas and Mike drive me back to Mum's on their way home. It is not too late to call a few of Mum's best friends, including Sam & Michael Milner, Laura & Adrian Cairns, "Splin" and others.

I have come to the point, this night, where I have no more tears left, nor can I talk anymore. It is time for me just to sleep. Magic dust would be good if it were possible tonight.

Chapter 6

I Speak with the Doctor

I contact the doctor first thing in the morning and ask many questions about all the possibilities and implications, everything that I couldn't think to ask at the time yesterday. It's not long before we are talking about the pros and cons of radiation treatment and chemotherapy. I have often heard that if the cancer doesn't kill you, the "chemo" will. The doctor explains that there are some circumstances which justify taking this direction. Mum's situation, however, is not one of them. He explains clearly the side effects of these therapies when directed to the brain. These treatments cannot do anything to allay her particular cancer. Then the one question I don't want to ask, but to which I need to know the answer: "How long does she have?" I ask. He replies, "I'm sorry. She only has six months to live. Perhaps a little more. She could always surprise us and continue for longer, though." I thank him for all he has done and for trying. I leave the office and head back to the apartment.

After careful and prayerful consideration, for Mum's own dignity and remaining quality of life, it seems that the best treatment we can offer is to get her home at some point and spoil her with love and care. We can do our best to make what time she has as comfortable and as meaningful as possible.

I make some calls to friends and to my work in the U.S. to tell them the news and the situation as it stands. It means that I am going to be here for at least six months and probably more. I'll be in touch as time moves on. In the meantime, there is going to be a lot to do here.

I make the trip on a bus back and forth to the hospital, which is on the other side of Bristol from Mum's flat. It sure beats walking that far! It is a dreary January even for England, cold and raining every single day. I stay all day every day. I get to know the tea ladies and other people who are visiting their loved ones. Why we make such a fuss over a hot beverage I'm not sure, but perhaps it's just something warm after the cold?

It is good to get over to Mum today. Understandably, she isn't on top of the world and isn't eating much. I encourage her and comfort her, and explain most of my conversation with the doctor. I explain about the differing treatments available, and how they are likely to make her feel and what the end result is likely to be. She takes all of this in and says, "Lee, I want to be home when I die. I don't want to die in pain or in a hospital." "Alright," I say. "Let's see what can be done, and there is talk about getting you home - so I think that's a good sign." She is pleased. We will wait and see how this is all going to turn out, and what the next step is to be in her care plan.

Her left side, although it has sensation, will not move or function well. But with some daily PT, there might be a full recovery. Continued therapy will be established at the BRI general hospital when she is moved there and it should help a great deal. This gives Mum a goal, to start thinking about getting proper use of her arm and leg again.

After a few more days, she has accepted her condition and the probable timescales involved. Emotionally, she seems to get stronger each day. She is really becoming herself again, and we laugh as I entertain her with stories of the green light discos.

Flowers arrive with dear friends Laura & Adrian Cairns, who come by to visit. Laura used to be a casting director, a singer and an actress. Adrian is an actors' trainer who also appears in films, a few shows and plays, and had a hand in training Sean Connery's son, Jason Connery. They are two wonderful and endearing people. Mum is a bit chattier as friends come over, enjoying their love and friendship. It seems odd, but she becomes a source of strength to them. They are more worried about Mum's situation than she is. She hugs her friends, tears flowing, and they feel encouraged by her positive spirit and peace of mind.

Michael and his wife Sam arrive later. Sam and Mum's history goes way back. She is probably Mum's longest standing friend of thirty something years. It is so good to see them, particularly after our recent 'phone conversation when I had to give them the bottom line concerning Mum's condition. They see each other and talk on the telephone fairly regularly. The news hit them pretty hard too.

They spend a good deal of time just sharing, crying, holding each other and hugging. Suddenly being faced with the imminent prospect of life's ultimate journey is a pretty confronting and emotional experience for anyone, especially hard when the dying person is oneself or a dearly loved friend.

Michael and I walk off to another waiting room, down the long corridor.

We put some change into a modern-looking, hot drink dispensing machine and receive a cup of "tea" which has the distinct flavor of used dishwater! Whatever made me think that a homemade cup of tea would come out of a hot drink machine. After his first sip, Michael's face indicates that he's drawn the same conclusion, and we both dispose of the full cups of hot "yuk" in the trashcan.

The following day it is evident that Mum is beginning to make some progress, being able to wiggle her left toes and to move her left hand increasingly. She is doing so well that the staff decide to move her into her very own room. It is used from time to time as the isolation unit, but there has been no one in here for a while. They decide it will work for Mum until she is moved to the BRI hospital closer to her home, literally a five-minute walk away for me.

A move into a wheelchair is a nice change and a great encouragement. Wow! What a difference a change in scenery can make after being stuck in bed for almost four weeks! Mum is feeling decidedly upbeat for certain. I wheel her slowly out of the ward and up part of the corridor and into the gift shop and back. Her strong pain medication is now being reduced and she is her usual full-of-life, cheery self. Under the circumstances that's quite amazing, I think!

"Well, here I am," I think. "Mum has approximately six months to live. My work and everything is back in the U.S. Should I even be thinking of this? Do I have a choice? What is most important?

Nothing, but *nothing*, is more important at this time than being here with Mum, and the circumstances are amazingly such that…well, I am able to be here, if I make the choice to stay. I can always get another job and find another home. Isn't life just a succession of choices really? I know what to do in this particular situation, anyhow. I have already made my choice."

Freedom, at last! As nice as this hospital has been, the BRI is just a short walk from Mum's flat. The only problem there is…CARDIAC Hill! Florida is nice and flat, but Bristol is like the Himalayas, and the sensation you feel after climbing this hill must be akin to that which you experience after scaling the peak of some sky bound mountain. It's so steep that some cars, especially in winter, can't even drive up to the top. No wonder they built a hospital right there!

It is a big move from the fine hospital and staff at Frenchay over to the Bristol Royal Infirmary. "Quality Street" sweets and thank you cards are in order for the nurses, along with photographs and a great deal of gratitude. This is a daily occurrence for these wonderful angels they call "nurses." They are simply not thanked or paid enough for all they do.

Mum is transferred to a BRI ward where she knows a couple of nurses. It is the same ward in which she collapsed almost a month ago. This is where her road to recovery will continue until she's regarded as fit enough to leave. After hugs from a few nurses, she is settled in nicely and obviously feels at home again straight away. She is glad that I don't have to make the late bus trips or that the neighbors do not have to come so far anymore. Always thinking of others!

~ ✚ ~

A Beautiful Journey

The new routine becomes established over the next few days. I return one morning after breakfast and draw near to Mum's bedside, noticing tears streaming down her cheeks. We hug for a while, saying nothing. As I lean back, she begins to tell me what is going on. She says that she has been feeling pretty calm generally, and then last night she had a vision that has left her with an amazing sense of peace. These are tears of joy, not sadness, Lee.

She describes it to me: *"I am in a long canoe, like a dugout. It is drifting slowly down the middle of this beautiful calm river. To either side is a green bank of reeds, grass, and flowers, and beyond that are trees. It is a sunny day with a clear blue sky and a few white puffy clouds. Straight ahead and far in the distance, I can see a soft, bright light at the end of the river. I am stretched out with my feet in front, leaning back against the chest of a man. He is softly stroking my head and my right shoulder and, with a calming soft voice, is telling me that I am safe and everything will be okay. As I slowly look up, I see a kind, strong, confident face smiling back. I feel so peaceful in his presence that I don't need to ask Him anything. I'm on a beautiful journey, Lee. When I close my eyes, His presence is right here, as if I can almost feel Him gently stroking my shoulder & head. Jesus doesn't look the way everyone thinks he looks."* With a warm smile and tears she says, *"Lee, I am at peace, complete peace..."*

"Wow! How incredible is that?" I exclaim, B-b-b." When did this happen? She says it started a little the previous night, but the feeling of peace is strong today.

I wonder at first whether the medication has affected her, but the medication she is on now are not anything that would give her delusions and, in my judgment, she is her normal self. This gives me too a sense of peace, that she possesses such an inner calm from this time onwards.

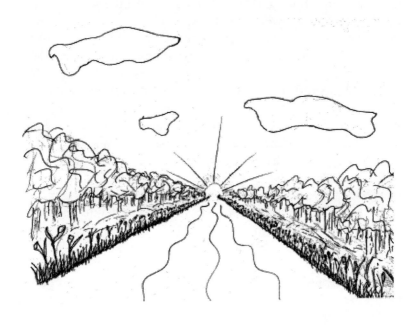

"A beautiful journey"

We catch up with what is going on in the town, and how I am coming along with the home projects. I ask Mum to confirm that it is bright PURPLE she wants in the bathroom, with white trim. "Yes," she says emphatically, and cork tile throughout the entire hall/passage area? "Yes, I'm certain that's what I want." "Okay then," I concede. "It'll all be done for when you arrive home."

I have painted before and commence taking everything out of the bathroom, preparing it for a good purple and white trim bathing all over. I manage to get some on the walls, some on the black and white tiled floor and the rest drips down my elbow. It dries fairly quickly, so I move everything back in. The next morning I inspect my handiwork and, as I look closer, I realize it needs a second coat! It is all done in another day. Bright purple! Hmmm!

I walk a short distance from Mum's to visit the Indian corner shop. As you walk in, the smell of curry doesn't so much tease your senses, it smacks you! The Indian video is playing in the VCR. The high-pitched voices and music are blaring. I think, "when in Rome, do as the Romans..." But how silly of me, we're in England! Everything in the shop has a fresh curry smell. I feel bad that I have to interrupt the shopkeepers' Indian film. They sigh. I flash money in front of them and that finally catches the attention of the proprietor and his wife. Life goes on and for them, the show must go on! I hope it has a happy ending.

After a few moments my sense of smell returns. Off I go back to the flat to tackle the new flooring and then to deliver these fine Indian goodies to Mum.

I sit by her, trying out the brand new airflow-seating-cushion-pad thing. At some point, when she is ready, they will maneuver her on to this chair. But I get to try it in the meantime.

We talk about life in the past, present, and future. She smiles as she reminisces about our last two weeks in India. "Can you believe some of the things we have had the opportunity to do, Lee?" she asks. "I know," I agree. "We have done a lot of fun things." "Can you fathom how we escaped from that compound in India?" she enquires, suddenly.

During our final two weeks back in Delhi, Mum had had the idea that it might be good to visit the older brother of the Guru who had so much inspired her life in recent years. She had heard there had been a miscommunication between the two brothers and since she was here, on the spot - so to speak - maybe *she* could sort of...help settle things between them.

She called the Guru's older brother, explaining who we were. He indicated that we should come and stay overnight while we were in Delhi. He said he would send his driver to pick us up at our hotel.

After quite a long drive we eventually arrived - not at a house, but a huge walled property. The driver pulled off the main road and stopped at the large entrance. He beeped the horn and a tiny square peep door opened. A face was peering to see who was there. It closed quickly, and the big double wooden gate opened to let the car in. It drove into what was a huge place, almost the size of a little town. It reminded me of an old Western film set. There were buildings on the left with the main building on the right. A few servants greeted us, but not the brother. He would meet us later at dinner, they said.

We were shown separate rooms to sleep in and we placed our luggage in Mum's room. One of the housekeepers, after pointing out a few things, suggested it would be more secure to leave our passports overnight in the house safe. We thought that would be a good idea and handed them over, together with our airline tickets. We were told that dinner was casual and would be served in a couple of hours in a building she pointed out. For now, though, we were to feel free to walk about the spacious grounds.

Mum was quite excited about all this, this being the family of the Guru and all! As we walked about, it seemed like a little town center. The buildings weren't made of wood but brick, covered in a thick layer of dust. The place had the distinct feeling of having seen better days, and was not used much anymore.

Nearly two hours later we arrived at the dinner area and began looking for the door into the dining room and the table. We noticed that people were beginning to sit down on the floor in the entrance hall. Perhaps dinner was going to be a long wait after all? They were a peaceable looking group mainly comprised of bald guys, mostly Indian, but there were a few Westerners apart from us, including a Scotsman, a young lady from America and a French couple with their baby. Others arrived and did the same as the earlier group and sat down. Two rows of people gradually took shape, sitting on the floor facing each other with about six feet in between. This evidently *was* the dining area!

All of a sudden a slight man came from the kitchen area with vegetables. They were hand-made circular banana leaves...oh! There plates. He placed one on the floor directly in front of each person. We sat, observed and copied what the others did. Then the doors opened and a few people came out with pots of rice and a yellow watery substance, called "Dahl," then a chapatti (a kind of unleavened bread) and stainless steel cups for water. With a ladle one man put a big blob of rice and then a big blob of the yellow substance on each leaf and then a chapatti. There were no knives, spoons or forks, so we watched with interest. You couldn't pick the leaf up without dropping your dinner on the floor.

After the last person was served, the people held a moment of silence and then began to eat. The man directly opposite dipped his right hand into the food, held his fingers together and, with one swift motion, his hand came up and placed the food in his mouth. Okay. Looks easy. We did the same... almost. Apparently I was given a leaky leaf, and my yellow blob was forming a little puddle. Mum was quite serious. She used the rice-perimeter-around-the-yellow-blob method. Her leaf wasn't leaking. She then broke off some chapatti and pinched the rice and yellow stuff together with it. She was obviously happy. Although my puddle was getting bigger, I continued trying to copy the man opposite me. I stuck my hand in, grabbed some of the blob and, as I raised my arm and got inches from my face, I flattened my hand out, as someone would feed a horse. I got some in my mouth, some on my face and some dripping down my arm. The kitchen door opened once more.

The man came out again (Mr. Blob), walked around and added more of the same to everyone's leaf for the second time.

I decided to go for the now well-tested rice-around-the-blob method and used the chapatti like a spoon. Towards the end of the meal the chap next to me demonstrated how to grab some rice, roll it into the dahl (making it half the size of a golf ball) then, pressing the fingers together, with the thumb behind the ball, lifting it to mouth level and gently flicking it in. I was happy for him, for his knowledge and his skill, but I still wanted to tell him about this invention we have in my country which we call "cutlery." Mum thoroughly enjoyed the meal. The brother was not there for dinner [I don't imagine sitting on the floor with leaking leaves eating white and yellow blobs was quite his thing.]

Nearly all the people at the property gathered with the brother later that evening, to hear him speak. As we approached the open floor seating area, we could see that he was already sitting. This was also when we first noticed the bodyguard, who came to his feet brandishing what looked like a rather large, heavy and long meat cleaver. The brother told his man to be at ease, and motioned us to come forward and sit. Then a few other Westerners approached, as did some of the people from dinner, so there were about thirty people gathered and sitting.

"Mr. Cleaver" made the announcement that if anyone approached the brother's room at night...well, it wouldn't be pretty, because he sleeps across the brother's doorway. I thought about saying "and it's been a pleasure to meet you too, sir!" But I held my tongue. We came to the conclusion that just in case Mr. Cleaver was in the habit of sleepwalking, we'd stay locked in our rooms at night.

To our great surprise, the brother began speaking by denouncing his younger brother as a fraud and claiming that it was *he* who was the *true* master and Guru.

We must all, he said, go out into the world to tell people this and make preparation for his arrival in the West. He told us we *must* follow his teachings over the next few weeks, and we couldn't leave these walls until we were considered "ready" to do this! I was thinking at this point that we must be on a film set, that somebody was about to yell, "Cut!" Well, the others certainly seemed to be good actors, but nobody yelled...

Some of the people moved forward and sweetly kissed his feet. Having just had dinner and no desire for dessert, we sat back and smiled at the others. After a few more words of enlightenment, the "true master" arose and left, with Mr. Cleaver following close behind. He was no doubt destined for a comfortable night's sleep, on the doorstep! Mum's expression said it all. She had evidently come to the conclusion that she had made a little mistake by suggesting to come here. No problem! We'd leave first thing in the morning. We would tell them we had...errr "The best sites of Delhi" bus tour booked; "we love the food, wonderful people! What a lovely place you have here, thanks ever so much, but we really need to go now,"... or something like that!

It was about three-thirty a.m. when I heard a knock on my door. I nearly swallowed my Adam's apple. OH NO! Was Mr. Cleaver sleepwalking?

Happily, it was only one of the bald guys from dinner. He told me it was time to meet and meditate in the circle room. It wasn't optional apparently, because he stood by my door waiting.

He said, "Bring your blanket," (I wanted to tell him that I was a big boy now and didn't need to carry my blankey anymore!) and led me back to the big room, where the incense was burning and a few candles shed barely a dim light across the room. The other men sat around wrapped in their blankets or with them over their heads, quiet and meditating. I sat completely still. I knew how to behave... just be like everyone else, although I did nod off a couple of times. These were all men here. I wondered if Mum was doing the same with the women. Probably so. Two hours later they all got up and I went wandering back to my room, dragging my blankey.

I met up with Mum at the "eating floor" by six-thirty a.m., ready for the breakfast blobs. She had the same bleary-eyed look that I did. She had already had enough and wanted to get going right away! We had breakfast and then went to find someone who would let us leave. We were told we couldn't leave here until the brother said we could. Mum had a panicked look. We walked off and reasoned that we didn't feel we were in any immediate threat or danger, other than the possibility of bumping into Mr. Cleaver during the night. We could pretend and just go along with it all and wait and see what happened.

After a week of pretending, nothing had happened - apart from early wakeups, more blobs and sitting to listen to the brother's nightly speeches. So we made a plan.

I would start holding my side and looking as though I was in pain for a couple of days, adopting the 'I-don't-feel-well' expression. Then, by the third day, I would begin doing the "I'm-in-a-lot-of-pain" routine whereby Mum, having been a nurse, would examine me in view of others and announce her diagnosis. She would declare I had acute appendicitis and that I needed to go to a British hospital immediately (We would have to fly there first, of course!). The plan went well and Mum convinced everyone of my serious condition.

The very next morning, while at breakfast, the brother came out to see us at the eating floor. We explained how we would, indeed, promote his teachings over and above his brother's. We went on to thank him for all that he was doing for the world and for blessing us with his presence and for showing us the way to the '*true* light' (He liked that one!)

Suddenly Mr. Cleaver appeared from nowhere. He looked characteristically stern as he approached our area at a brisk pace, the long meat cleaver dangling from his belt. He stopped suddenly in front of us, quickly reaching inside his jacket. We held our breath. I dropped a blob, and he pulled out …our passports and flight tickets!

The house servants helped pack our bags and bring them to the car. Mum said goodbye, and I… continued with a convincing moan and a pathetic smile. It wasn't long before the compound disappeared into the background, and an hour later the airport loomed in front of us. We thanked the driver and he drove away. The brother's staff had apparently called the airport and airline ahead of us and, when the airline staff saw our tickets, they took us out of line and whisked us to a nice waiting area away from the madness.

We still held on to our cause and wouldn't let up until we were safely on the plane and in the air.

It was three hours later when the clunk of the undercarriage signaled that we were finally in the air and on our way home. We smiled and hugged in celebration, but quietly, so as not to attract attention - and Mum let out tears of relief.

From the window we could see that the sun was beginning to go down on the dry, hot, barren land. We'd *never* forget our trip to India!

Sitting up in the hospital bed, Mum says she is feeling so much better emotionally that she wants me to contact her friends and neighbors. She wants me to give them the scoop on what's happened and to tell them they can come and visit. Her left side is moving slightly, but there is no real strength in her arm or leg. She can wiggle her toes. The physical therapist has indicated that at some point they hope to get her on a walking frame, if she can make further progress.

Today's mission is to get her a new stereo CD/tape/radio boom box for her bedside. I think it'll liven things up around here. I'll get headphones just in case the other patients are not as enthusiastic. Mum's music taste spans classical, reggae, smooth jazz, Andrea Bocelli, contemporary spiritual and much besides and in between - "eclectic," I think, is the best description. I'll focus upon the more mellow things she likes for now, especially material with uplifting, encouraging lyrics, plus anything else that she wants. How amazing to look at Mum today! In many ways you wouldn't think anything was wrong with her. She is such a cheerful soul. This all seems so surreal, but I'm here and it is not a dream. I'd better get into town and find a music system.

Outside, isn't it odd how the world just keeps going on as if nothing else is of any concern? How *can* everyone seem so cheerful, when so much tragedy is happening with Mum? My Mum is *dying*! That surely is at least newsworthy! It *can't* be just another day for all!

Each person's life has his or her own circumstances and tragedy. Someone else's parent, child, relative or close friend is in a situation just like mine, or worse. But these are our circumstances, and it is important to me and my mum, regardless of other peoples' pains, lesser or greater as they may be. The world will not stop. People will be laughing and life, regardless of anyone or anything, marches forward… relentlessly.

[It is truly not *what* happens to you in life but *how* you deal with it that is important.] I commit to making this the most comfortable time possible for Mum in any way I can.

The English catalog shop! Where would life be without the catalog shops? Long gone are the hunting days for sure! We are reduced to looking through a picture catalog book, picking a number. Yeah, but which number? Okay, so I have to go back and search again. I wrote the page number! Add the extra insurance... should I or shouldn't I? It's always more money, more money.

This thing has a CD, radio, tape and a base-booster-something-button, too... that means you can annoy anyone for miles! With the headphones included, the system sounds like a good one to me. Nothing discreet about where you bought this, though. The huge plastic carrying bag has the catalog company logo all over it (Look everyone! This man bought this pretty cheap. He could have bought a better quality system had he more money, but he hasn't... Just to let you know!).

Mum's eyes glisten with excitement as I walk into the ward looking like Father Christmas. I unwrap, unpack and set up the CD player by her bedside, as others look over. There she sits with her headphones on and the music going. She blissfully and tearfully smiles. She can now get lost in the music, temporarily escape into her own little world. Relief at last, from the incessant noise of beeping equipment and general daily hum of activity going on around her! It can't be easy just to lie here, day in, day out.

Hopefully (God Willing), she'll be walking and will have some independence soon. I'll bring more of her relaxing music over tomorrow, I decide.

Chapter 7

Contacting her sister

During this introspective time, Mum realizes that she wants to attempt (while she is still able) to set right certain emotionally difficult situations that exist in her life. Some of them are with her sisters and she asks me to contact "Aunt Marion" first. They haven't been in touch for nearly twenty years. That implies a lot of hurting! Mum is ready to accept that she doesn't really remember what their quarrels or misunderstandings were about. Many years have passed; even if she could remember, it is all "water long under the bridge" at this point. I'll make the call when I arrive home later.

I am a little nervous myself about calling Aunt Marion, but - here goes! I call her in London, about one hundred miles away. A bubbly voice comes on the line. I explain who I am and, with a gasp on the other end, she said she recalls seeing me as little, cute and cuddly. I assure her that, actually, I haven't changed much...I'm just bigger! It doesn't take long to get to the topic of Mum. When she asks the question "And how is Baby?" (Mum's childhood nickname), she listens in stunned silence as I bring her up to date. Without my asking, she wants to drive over as soon as possible. We arrange for Saturday this weekend after lunch. She hangs up after some sweet words of encouragement.

I give Mum the news first thing in the morning when I arrive at the hospital. She is so pleased and wants to know every word that was shared. I manage to convey the headlines of the conversation.

As men, we seem to do fine with a nod and a grunt, while women want every little detail. Oh well, *"vive le difference!"* I suppose.

The next few days pass in great anticipation, during which time Mum has, apparently, become the unofficial ward guard. From her vantage point, she manages to signal to the nurses when one patient decides to light up a cigarette while in bed next to the oxygen outlet! The patient puffs away, smiles and kindly offers the nurse one, as the nurse approaches her... like a heat-seeking missile!

Mum also manages to notify the nurses when another lady across from her wanders off twice in her nightdress, not knowing where she is going, why, how or even *who* she is. She is brought back safely, insisting that she is now ready for the shopping expedition... After frequenting the ward often, it is noticeable how many people are not visited very much by anyone: So, when Mum has an abundance of flowers, fruit or chocolates on any given day, she shares them with others who are less fortunate.

On Saturday I start the day with the usual weekend energy of most people who are happy to be anywhere other than work. Mum is up early, too.

When I arrive she has a special bath organized and a hairdresser is on her way over. So I go to town for a couple of hours to take care of some administrative duties for Mum.

I am surprised at the number of beggars asking for money. They are mainly young people in their mid thirties, some younger and a few older. Many of them seem to have a dog in tow. The new fashion seems to be to have a pet, since people feel sorry for the sad looking dog and are more willing to give the beggar money. There are government benefit advantages to this arrangement in England too, I've heard. At the same time an unconditionally loving pet, can be a real comfort too.

I'm back at the BRI before long. Mum takes this opportunity to notify me that her toenails need attention. At first I suggest putting the sheet over them. She is diabetic and so cutting her nails is a delicate business. She informs me the nurses are not allowed to perform such a duty. I tackle it confidently and quickly, and she still had ten toes when I am finished. Pointing to the red nail polish she asks, "Would you, please?" Well, I've painted a fence, some doors and walls before but this is a much smaller area. After so many years, I suppose she wants to look her very best. I manage to get some on her toe, lots in between the toes and some on her sheet. Mum squints with her glasses on, can see red from her end of the bed, and that is that! A job well done! I'm hoping her sister will stay at the talking end and not look down here. Mum's hair is growing well and the hairdresser has been able to cover up the scar on her head so that it is not so obvious, which pleases Mum no end. A quick clean up, clear up and I'm done! She is all ready to meet her public!

An hour or two later I hear a commotion at the entrance and see four people surveying the ward from the doorway. I notify Mum they have arrived, and she asks how she looks. "Great, Mum. You look great!" I reassure her. I recognize her sister from photos as my Auntie Marion, and I beckon all of them to come in. They recognize my features just as I recognize theirs. I know the tall man to be my young cousin, Jay, from another aunt. The other two are Aunt Marion's children, Stephanie and Marco. They all proceed forward, a lovely looking group of people. We embrace in a long hug while I think of all the lost time and missed opportunities. (After so much time, why does it always take something as final as this for people to look past their differences and move forward? The reasons are vast and many. I'm just glad that, even at this late stage, Mum and Marion have a little time to make their peace with one another.)

We all stand back as Mum and her sister look into each other's eyes for a silent moment. Searching for common ground in a smile, perhaps. They find it in tears - representing the loss of so *many* years, which begin streaming down both their faces. They reach out to each other hugging, kissing and crying, wiping tear's from each other's faces.

I hug my three younger cousins. There isn't much to say right now. We all let our emotions bridge the long separation in silence.

Mum acknowledges and kisses the three younger family members. The cousins and I sit together and Marion sits by Mum, holding Mum's hand. They talk & talk as if no one else were here. We don't interrupt them.

My one younger cousin, Jay, is now six feet three inches tall, the other two cousins are less than six feet. All three are dear, sweet people and I feel that I've missed out over the years by not knowing them. We have unmistakably similar features; dark hair, chiseled jaw lines and pronounced dark eyebrows. We definitely look related. The small talk gets underway; we discuss what each of us is doing now, and when we last remember even seeing one another. My sister walks in with her husband and once again we all meet and greet. I suppose in some sense we are family. Yet we are complete strangers. Sad, but in this case it is true. I suggest tea and walk with Jay to get some refreshments for all of us. The nurse comes by and is happy to see Mum with so many loving people around her. The nurses, too, are excited about Mum's sister coming. She has told them it has been many years since they have seen each other. Mum looks good and feels good. I can see it is a wonderful day for her.

The daylight dwindles, and all too soon it is time for them to leave and head back to London. We exchange promises to see each other again or, if a chance arrives, I will visit them in London over a weekend while I'm in England. We all hug our goodbyes. I walk them to the ward entrance and, giving a final wave, bid them a safe journey home as they depart down the corridor.

It has been a wonderful and emotional day for Mum. She is elated to have had this time and the opportunity it offered, but she is exhausted now. She mentions how wonderful it was to see them and say hello, though it was really... goodbye. They speak to each other on the phone often from that day onwards.

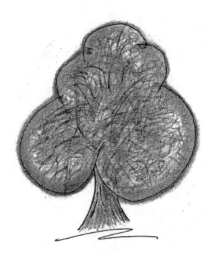

Chapter 8

A visit from the physical therapist

As the news gets around, friends and neighbors come from near and far to visit, and the phone almost rings off the hook for Mum. Of course no one gets a personal phone line, and the staff have to keep handing the wireless phone over from the main nursing station on the ward. The system seems to work well, though, and they do not seem bothered by bringing it over as much as they do.

The physical therapy people visit again. Having done what they have up to this point, they sense that Mum has already reached her optimum level of ability. She has some feeling in her arm and leg, but neither can function. The experts have come to the conclusion that there is nothing more they can do to help Mum: They give the news to the head nurse. She beckons me over. She sits me down and explains the limited options for Mum's future.

The fact now is painfully clear that Mum is paralyzed on her left side because of the damage done by the tumor. Inside I feel wrenched about what to do. The nurse continues to explain that, when Mum is discharged from the hospital, she can't be home alone. This means her going to a nursing home unless someone is going to stay with her twenty-four hours a day, seven days a week...until the inevitable.

The news of her left side will filter through more subtly to Mum as it becomes increasingly apparent to her that she cannot do the exercises. However, in the best of spirits, she tells me how she is looking forward to going home soon.

"Who could possibly do this?" I ask myself. My sister lives sixty miles away and has to work full time. It is way too much to put on Mum's friends and neighbors. There is no other immediate family member now, and that only leaves...*me*. Oh wow! Mum is happily unaware of the decisions being made on her behalf at this time. Life will have to go on hold regardless of the pile I'll have to deal with when I get back to Tampa. There are priorities in life that we just have to get in order. I may have prioritized a lot of things from back to front over the years, but at least this is one priority I've got in its *proper* order.

A few days later, a meeting is held and I am asked to be there along with a district nurse, hospital nurse, physical therapist, social worker and hospital administrator. We are all in a cramped nurses' office to discuss Mum. After all the introductions are made, the hospital nurse leads the way by going over Mum's present and expected condition. She indicates that Mum is doing very well under the circumstances and that she expects her to be discharged within the next three weeks. Hence, the meeting to decide the care plan and the next step. The district nurse asks me what my thoughts are for Mum after discharge. I indicate I plan to take her home, since that is what she would like. She then asks me who will be caring for her. Errr... "That will be me!" I announce.

Without painting a rosy picture, the district nurse goes on to inform me about what exactly will be involved in caring for Mum and what I will be expected to do all day, every day, for at least six months or more. It's as if this information might weaken my resolve, but it is mainly to give me a blunt and clear idea of what I am letting myself in for. Having explained everything in painful detail, she then asks whether I am prepared to do this. I reply "Yes, I most certainly am." In response, she smiles with a look that seems to say: "you-poor-poor-dear; you-have-no-clue-what-is-in-store!" But I tell her that I am willing to do all of that and more. These few, but determined, words really start the conversations going.

The different departments start to engage each other and inform me of the various grants and assistance that will be available to Mum. The equipment needed, the medications, the nurse rota, the care helpers, etcetera and etcetera. To my relief, I realize that at least I am not going to be left entirely alone in this undertaking. We all exchange handshakes as they agree to keep in contact and discussion, and to inform me about what steps need taking next as the situation develops.

Even though I am going into this with my eyes wide open, it is all still new and quite intimidating. But the bottom line here is that Mum has some time left, and we will make that time as comfortable and warm as possible for her. She has always known she is loved and cherished by many. [Ultimately, all we ever want as humans is simply to be loved and accepted.]

I will take one step at a time, as that's how we get through many of our journeys in life; and before you know it, a lot of ground is covered. I think the mental step here is the biggest one. To a larger degree, this is one small step in life and a giant leap of faith for me.

I am thinking about many things as I face the decisions that need to be made. What about my job, my car, and my accommodation? I am not yet at a point with the company whereby my absence will shatter the United States' economy. The saying is that graveyards are full of indispensable people, but somehow the world manages to go on without them. I am staying with friends and most of my things are in storage. My car is paid for, and the remaining bills can be covered. A friend reminds me of a verse in the Bible - Romans 8:28 (KJV); it is uncanny and seems to me to capture this whole situation somehow: "And we know that God causes all things to work together for good…"

What of these "things" to which the passage alludes? They are but circumstances if you like. My own current situation can be seen as extraordinary, as I do have the opportunity to make the necessary commitment at this particular juncture in life. Do I stay and care for Mum, or is everything else a priority? I do not have any other responsibilities, so for me it is a relatively uncomplicated consideration and sacrifice. I am able to choose to care for Mum. I have the sense that I need to be here, not out of duty but out of love for a dear friend and a precious Mum. It is more of a privilege and an honor than a sacrifice. Oh, without the shadow of a doubt, this is not going to be a walk in the park either...

I think of the movie title, "Sleepless in Seattle." Mine might be called "Clueless in Bristol!" I muse, wryly. I know that I am really flying by the seat of my pants here and making commitments that, at this point in time, I am not sure how I am going to be able to fulfill. But in my heart I know I must be here. I'm scared that I may not be able to do all that needs to be done. I remember a saying that impressed me when I was a boy: "failure is not an option." This would be a good motto for me to adopt!

The official inspection

First of all there needs to be an inspection of Mum's place to allow the doctors in charge to move in all the medical equipment. The inspection is to be done the following day and, based on the result, the authorities will give the go-ahead (or not) for Mum to come home when they judge it to be the right time.

I know that there are some things to prepare, and I am not sure really about the room size for maneuverability. As I arrive at the flat and look around, I realize that Mum's bedroom is simply too cramped: But there is a lot of furniture in the more spacious front room. It also has a smooth shiny new wooden floor, with plenty of natural light. Hmmm, well-this will have to be it then! I drag all the furniture out and squeeze it in and around what is now my bedroom; it looks more cramped than ever in here now. I try to make it look as close to a home for me as I can, but it still ends up looking like a dump! Oh well...covering everything with sheets will have to suffice for now.

The inspector arrives the following day. It is one of the physical therapists, a sweet young Scottish lady. She isn't too sure about the bathroom color, but she likes the new flooring in the hallway. I still have glue on my fingers from doing that job! She doesn't go into my bed-dump-room since I have said the front room is where Mum will be. She is happy with that arrangement. Then she gives the kitchen a once over. After twenty minutes of house safety rules, commitment questions and filling out forms, she smiles and agrees to go ahead and approve the home suitable for patient and equipment. "Whoooopeeeeee!" I think to myself, and thank her very much. This is brilliant news and I will be so pleased to share it with Mum. It will really put her at ease, in as much as it can, concerning future plans. I imagine that, for most people, the opportunity to be at home at such a time would be very special- certainly, for Mum, this is the case.

As I walk into the hospital ward and see Mum, she has a disappointed look on her face and points to the CD player. At a quick glance, the crack is evident. The carry handle is askew and the aerial (antenna) has apparently decided to go in its own direction, indicating that gravity got the better of the CD player. I quickly explain that, at the last minute, I took out a small replacement policy. Not to worry! It is easy to see, from her big smile, that this news makes Mum very happy. Apparently she had gone to adjust the volume and the player wanted to meet the floor and leapt off the table. Have you ever seen the size of those little tables by the beds?

I share the news excitedly with Mum-that her home meets the hospital requirements, and that this means she can come home as soon as she is allowed to leave here. With more smiles and tears, she expresses her relief.

I wrap up the broken CD player. Walking out, I attempt the hill and go back to the catalog store. I find one at about the same price with a few more whistles and bells. At the exchange counter, I produce the receipt with coverage.

Two different supervisors examine the paperwork as though I had recently printed it myself. They keep looking up at me and back at the receipt, as if trying to identify me with a picture. Eventually, with raised shoulders and a nod, I get the executive approval to exchange. The new machine comes in a slightly bigger box, which means an enormously BIG bag. I reflect that this one would come in handy if I were on a sailboat and the main sail were to disappear during a voyage. I'd bring the bag out and hoist it up. I wonder whether I can get some sort of advertising fee for carrying this thing around? Hurrying back, I set up the new system and find some additional use for Scotch tape - that player isn't going anywhere now!

The day seems fairly busy for Mum, with visits from nurses and doctors throughout the day. The nurses seem ever vigilant concerning liquid consumption and food intake, and Mum is pretty good at keeping up her intake most of the time. I say most of the time because, although I'm sure the hospital food meets all the nutritional guidelines, it lacks excitement to the taste buds for her, and Mum loves her food. Consequently, Indian takeaways are often the order of the day. When you boil it all down to her activity level: food, water, music and company are all that is going on. Even a scenery change might do wonders for the spirit; the only scenery she has is Gurty across the room in the other bed, who keeps getting up and walking off.

Interesting visitors come and go... I get used to hearing silly questions, and things I haven't thought about previously but now know. Here are some examples of bedside conversations:

Question: "How are you?" Answer: "Very sick!"
Question: "How is the food?" Answer: "You try some and tell me!"
Question: "How long will you be here?" Answer: "Until they let me go home!"
Question: "Isn't there anything that can be done about it?" Answer: "A miracle!"

Stories abound of very sick friends who have Mum's same ailment! Or stories of how "I had a family member/friend, or my uncle's friend's brother's half cousin-in-law, whose wife's friend's sister had an auntie and her next door neighbor died of the same thing."

People seem to be clueless about what to say. I think they just get nervous and blurt out whatever comes into their head. This is often what happens when someone engages the jaw without first telling the brain. I come to the conclusion that people feel that if they can kind of relate to someone with a particular illness or situation by telling their own similar stories, somehow this puts them on the same wavelength as the patient. It doesn't! And even if it did, an unwell person in the bed doesn't need to hear about all this extra stuff, because he or she already has enough going on. I should have put a sign up to remind people that silence is still considered golden. I find that friends or visitors feel awkward in the silence of a moment and feel bad, sad and just plain helpless really to do anything.

The sense of being powerless is a strong one. As humans we will try to do almost *anything* to give someone's life a chance. This sense is understandably exaggerated when it's someone who's very close to us, and because we are in the twenty-first century with all the advances in medical technology, and yet sometimes there is nothing that can be done.

A hug, a handclasp and a prayer for comfort and peace definitely seem to be the better options if the visitor has nothing to say, and then just to convey to the patient and family that help is available as, where and when it's needed.

The days pass with many visits to the hospital. The routine is quite straightforward. I wake fairly early and climb around the furniture to get clothes from my suitcase. I only brought enough clothes for a couple of weeks... I have a lovely "cuppa" (hot-cup-of-tea) and get organized. I wander off to the shop, pick up a snack or prune juice for Mum, and walk down to the BRI. I head along the corridor to the lift, which takes me up to the fourth floor.

I turn right along another corridor, take a second lift to the seventh floor, walk down one more corridor and I'm in the ward! There are five beds along the left wall, in between narrow windows, and the same on the right. Mum is in the last bed on the right, next to the nurses' station.

Beyond the nurses' station, there are another five or so beds lined up in a similar fashion on either side. The colors are all quite neutral and the room is well lit, with overhead fluorescent lights dangling from the twelve-foot ceilings.

Mum's first question after a hug is, "Have you had breakfast yet?" Then she makes suggestions about good places to go. We chat a while as she explains how her night went. The patients' sleep is often interrupted during the fairly quiet, but still busy, nightshift. The tea lady arrives on her rounds, offering tea and biscuits. She fills Mum's no-spill beaker.

I opt to go down to the cafeteria. Having arrived at the ground floor level, I now walk into the well-lit and busy hospital pedestrian tunnel, which goes under the road and connects to the next hospital, and enter the much-spoken-about hospital café. The English café...now, that is a unique experience! Where else can you get a healthy British breakfast consisting of fried bread, baked beans, bacon, fried eggs, stewed tomatoes, fried black pudding (clotted pigs' blood wrapped in a sausage skin), toast, jam and tea? After eating all of that, it is just as well that you are at the hospital, and - please wait before attempting the hill! I just order toast & tea. It is a busy café, full of nurses, doctors and many visitors. I quickly finish up and head back through the tunnel.

Keeping Mum company is fine. We talk about many things, from the past to the present and everything in between, including our travel adventures of the past. As I have said it was in India that we became very good friends, and from that time forward we developed a unique bond. Mum was a young mum in her attitude and outlook. She loved to laugh, and can recall many stories and fond memories. As a kid, I would often do impersonations and could do them of nearly anyone. It wouldn't take much to get her into fits of laughter. This *often* got me out of trouble quicker than I had gotten into it!

Mum is recalling two American comedy guys, Cheech and Chong. I do my part, trying to get the American Los Angeles Spanish accent, along with the scene she has in mind. I'm getting into the groove with my hands moving, my arms swinging, and I've got the head thing going. She begins howling with laughter. I know that I must be looking crazy right about now. As I turn, the guests visiting the patient next to Mum are staring with their mouths open. I'm sure they have only two thoughts…will their mother be safe here tonight, and *when* will this man be given his next dose of medication?

There are days when we do not say much. Just being here is good, and we don't always have to talk just to talk. Sometimes I sit in the comfy chair next to her bed, lean back, and drift off to sleep as well.

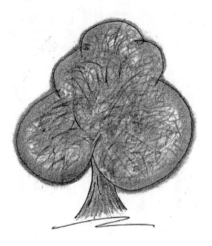

Chapter 9

The equipment arrives

Because of the distance, losing immediate touch with close friends feels problematic for me. I miss the daily communication with them. I use internet cafes as often as I can. I'm surprised by how popular these places are in England. I manage to get a few notes out to friends, letting them know what's going on here. It is so good to receive an encouraging e-mail message from a friend, or even a simple card.

I wasn't raised in Bristol. Mum moved here nearly fourteen years ago because she had friends here and liked the area. Being in an unfamiliar city takes a little getting used to at first. But I am finding my way around now and getting used to the smallness of it all compared to the U.S. I'm getting used to the different shopping hours, and where the best shops and bargains are. As each day passes I awaken to the fact that, as unbelievable as this all seems to be, it is for real. It is odd, too, as time goes on, that I invariably receive a call from one of Mum's friends who perhaps has been away and has no idea about events these last few weeks. Each one is overwhelmed with the news. I seem to be learning how best to encourage her tearful and deeply saddened friends, as they suddenly learn of Mum's terminal condition.

Mum is such a cheerful soul; you wouldn't think anything was the matter at first. It is amazing how she is calming to others, even as she is at peace with herself and what is happening. It is special to have her friends come from afar, just to be here for part of the day, and then go all the way home.

It is good for Mum to be on the receiving end now of love and attentiveness, having given to others for so much of her life!

I get her a take-away curry for dinner, which she enjoys immensely. The alternative would have been tonight's special serving of mashed mush with boiled mush. It didn't look appetizing to me either (Though quite nutritious, of course!) The nurse explains that Mum's increasing appetite is due to her being on a steroid, which she takes to keep down the swelling inside her head. One side effect is a big appetite. Of all the side effects to have to have, this is a joyous one for Mum. She loves her food!

The NHS (National Health Service) and community nursing services contact me at Mum's home to arrange delivery of the special equipment we will need in order to nurse Mum here. The front room is clear of everything, and first to arrive is a brand new electric hospital bed on wheels, complete with a special air mattress cover, which moves in slow ripples to help prevent bedsores from developing. The deliverymen set it all up. We position the bed opposite the window, where Mum can enjoy plenty of sunlight. We do get sunshine in England, on occasion-I have seen it in a picture in the National Geographic Magazine. I sign the paperwork the men leave, and I stare at all the equipment. Happy that Mum will have her wish to come home, I feel scared for a moment...almost overwhelmed. I know that somehow I can do whatever it is I'm going to be called upon to do.

Over the next few days, all the equipment is set in place. The oddest piece is the electric lifter, which reminds me of the three-wheeled v-base shape of the equipment used to remove car engines. As Mum is quite limited in the use of her own body, in order to enable her to go to the bathroom, she must be maneuvered on the bed so as to be positioned into a sling. The lift arm lowers, attaches to the sling strap ends, lifts her out of her bed, lowers her into the wheelchair, detaches from the lift arm and then is wheeled to the little room. The wheelchair has a special seat, which is much like a toilet seat. The entire wheelchair slides over the toilet backwards. Then the reverse needs to happen in order to put her back to bed. This ritual must be repeated three times everyday, and takes two people to coordinate.

I lower the lift arm down, sit myself in the sling, hook it up and then lean back almost completely flat on the floor. I hold the remote control and press the up button. The arm slowly takes up the slack and the strain as it lifts me off the floor; an odd sensation, but it works well and swivels about. As long as I don't get stuck swinging in the air by myself and calling for help, I'll be okay. Fortunately, it works fine.

By means of a handheld controller, the bed can be raised or lowered to the floor, and the back of the bed can be raised or lowered from a flat position to bring the patient into an upright position of any angle.

The air mattress pump equipment works well and is silent in its operation twenty-four hours a day. It simply attaches and hangs independently from the end of the bed, supplying air to the mattress cover.

A special chair is brought in for the times when Mum will want to sit up in a comfy chair, rather than be in bed. This will depend on her having the strength to feel able to do so. It is a maroon, high backed electronic chair, which can rise to stand a patient upright or be reclined until almost horizontal. It could be my new favorite chair. "I'd better try it out, just in case something isn't working right!" I tell myself. I decide to try it a few more times, just to be sure.

A knock on the door reveals a friendly and confident nurse, Julie, who is in charge of the nurses for this district. She explains about the medication: all the pills Mum needs, when they are prescribed, how I reorder them and the timeframe within which to do this so as not to go short. She gives me emergency numbers, doctors' numbers and contact information for the social services. At this point, she explains that I will have help three times each day at 08:00 a.m., 1:30 p.m. and 7:30 p.m., when caregivers will take care of Mum's personal needs. I'll need to help with the lift equipment and maneuvering, which I'm more than happy to do. This is a great relief, as I had thought this was all just for me to do. Julie also explains that a nurse will be coming each morning for the initial week to check Mum's vital signs, and then every other day, and that the doctor will be in once a week and then can be called as needed. She proceeds to ask about my "meal plans."

Hmmm; I have been wondering how I will manage to produce the variety of meals that will be required. As brilliant as I am at toast and tea and bowls of Cornflakes, I somehow know that this limited repertoire would not quite give Mum the variety of food necessary, and I've already reflected that I must avoid burning the salad at all costs! So, having no time to lose, I went out to buy a cookbook, and now only need to learn to cook. I chose one written by Jamie Oliver, the popular young British chef. I have seen him on TV and he makes cooking look fun rather than a chore, and creates simple but exotic looking dishes (I'm thinking of the "simple" part). I could do a few easy meals and salads to begin with, and fetch in an Indian takeaway on Saturday nights to add variety. So I tell Julie that, yes, indeed I have started planning meals! She indicates that all will be coordinated and prepared for Mum's arrival by ambulance in three days' time.

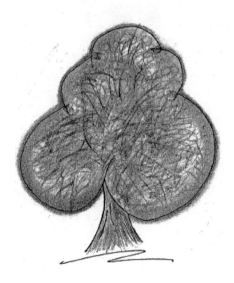

Chapter 10

Home at last

Mum is most excited about the prospect of coming home at this point! She has been grateful for all she has had done for her in the hospital, and the great kindness extended by the nurses and staff, but now it is time for home; for her to rest away from the hustle and bustle of the hospital groove.

She asks for more chocolates to be delivered to the nurses' station, and "thank you" cards for them all. They will miss being spoiled with chocolates! I take a trip into town and come across noisy demonstrators holding pictures of Bush and Blair and shouting about news of the present climate of events in the Middle East. I arrived at the conclusion long ago that there will always be people who are for or against anything based on what it can, or can't, do for them. I avoid the handouts and stop further up the street to listen to a street musician who is happily playing away a classical ditty on her violin. I drop a pound into her box and she gives me a nod. Was that a nod meaning "thank you," or "drop in another?" I smile and move off in my hasty search for chocolates and cards. I approach the small mall -or "arcade," as it is called here. I arrive at the place where I have previously found big boxes of Mum's favorite assorted chocolates, "Quality Street," and purchase two.

After eating all of these, those nurses will have to run for miles to get the weight off. Come to think of it, they probably burn it off right there, as they are rarely sitting down. Bless 'em...always on the go! I take the chocolates straight home and avoid the temptation to test them, only for quality assurance purpose of course. During the next day I make sure I get all the names, and write out cards to give when Mum leaves.

The big morning dawns and I arrive early. Mum is all smiles and full of excitement. The nurses have obviously become quite attached to her. They are all fussing around her. Lunchtime comes and extra portions are given. After dessert the mandatory cup of tea is served and, no sooner than precisely the moment planned, two ambulance attendants and their wheeled transport stretcher come into the ward. After clearing with the nurses' station exactly who is to be taken where, with confident smiles they approach Mum's bedside, together with two nurses who assist in making sure the change from bed to stretcher goes well. There are kind words expressed, hugs, kisses, waves, and tears as Mum is wheeled out of the ward. I say thank you to the nurses' station and leave the cards and chocolates from Mum, grab the last load of her personal items and head home for the five-minute walk, to arrive ahead of the ambulance.

It is a bright day with no rain in sight and a wonderful day for Mum to arrive home. The ambulance has had to take the one-way road system around, so I arrive back a couple of minutes before it does.

On arrival the attendants maneuver the transport stretcher, feet first, so Mum is able to see her garden as they wheel her down the garden path. She is excited to see what is growing and comments about some plants and her rose bush. She is then negotiated three steps down to the front door of her garden flat.

She notices the new cork-tiled floor I have laid, and likes the look of it. The attendants rest her stretcher next to her new bed, secure all wheels and position the equipment as it needs to be. I hold her head and, with one swift movement, we slide Mum from the stretcher to her bed. With the safety sides up, the catheter bag in its holder and the bedcovers up, the transporters back their way out, bidding us a last goodbye…the front door closes and, then, silence! No beeps, no hospital noises, no sense of being in the middle of a mall; just… quiet!

Mum lets out a loud, "Wow! I can't believe it! I'm home! Lee, for a while there I didn't think it was going to happen!" She calls me over, just wanting to hug, and to say thank you for making it possible to come home, and for just being here to help her through all this. She is so happy! Her smile and tears say it all! She asks about the garden, her friends and her neighbors.

I hand her the bed control, which is just like the one in the hospital, and also the stereo and TV controls. I step into the kitchen and put the tea on, and then proceed to unpack her bags and put her items away. The kettle starts to boil as the doorbell rings. Through the smoked French glass front door one can see it is a nurse. It is the head district nurse, Julie. She comes in with a big smile, wanting to know how Mum's move went. She wants to make sure all is as it needs to be, and to explain the procedures from today onwards. I introduce her to Mum, and they chat while I make us all a cup of tea.

Julie goes over the times with me that assistants (caregivers) will come.

Their job is to take care of Mum's personal needs three times a day, typically at 08:00 a.m., 1:30 p.m., and 7:30 p.m., she reiterates. I will help the person with the equipment, and getting Mum in and out of it. She covers the medications, and reviews all that I have collected from the pharmacy, when to order refills and the administration of the drugs. I suppose it is the bewildered look on my face that prompts her to suggest that she will bring back a medication box, which I can fill for a week at a time. We go over telephone numbers once again, and stress the fact that I am to have the cell phone with me at all times.

She is happy with all of this. I give Mum her tea. She now just wants to relax and watch some TV, at which point Julie asks me to sit with her in the kitchen. We leave Mum and close the kitchen door. Julie wants to be sure I am coping alright and that I am not feeling overwhelmed. She explains that this is what she does full-time, and she finds generally that it's not easy with one family member doing all that needs to be done. I assure her that I am fine, and will be okay, but if not I will let her know. With that answer she seems reassured all would be well. She says that she or one of her team will be in every morning this first week, anyhow, and they can carry on for longer if necessary until they feel the routine is stable and the caregivers are settled in their role.

She stops back in to check Mum and to check the catheter bag. She decides that the catheter bag is too small. It is really only a transport bag. She pulls out of her kit a proper-size bag and, with gloves on, unclips the old and clips on the new. Done! She cleans up, wishes us both well and reminds me to call anytime, twenty-four hours a day, if I need anything, even if I just have a question to ask. With that, she leaves the flat.

I am pleased that she came, and feel encouraged by her words. I don't feel entirely alone in this endeavor anymore.

It is time to sit for a moment and relax with Mum. No need to run back and forth, up and down the hill to the hospital or to the city center. I can just rest. Mum is quite happy with whatever has been arranged and asks me just to take care of everything as she doesn't want to have to think about any of it. Last year when I was here for three weeks helping her with the lung cancer treatments she suggested that, in case anything happened, she would like me to be able to have access to her small bank account. So we went to her bank and she added my name to her account. This is the type of event we'd envisaged, and our actions then have given me the freedom to take care of her bills now, whenever I need to. She doesn't have a great deal of income because she lives mostly on government subsistence. Two years previously, we also took care of a small life insurance policy, called a "final expense policy." It pays out just enough to take care of such an expense.

Mum said, "I trust you will do whatever is best, and I know your heart is in the right place." We both agreed at the time, and that was that.

I am glad we did this forward planning. Having done so proves to be a comfort to us now. Mum can relax, and so can I. She leans back and goes to sleep as I lie back in the soft chair and drift off too.

"Lee, what's for dinner?"…is the waking question, followed with "Can I have some tea?" "A curry, and "yes!" to the tea," is my answer. I have arranged for a nice Indian takeaway as her celebratory homecoming meal. "Oh great, thank you …When?" she asks. "Should be here by 6:00 pm." "Any snacks?" "Yep, you have a selection of Indian crunches, fruit, cheese and biscuits, or I can cook something if none of that appeals." "Some Indian crunch mix would be nice…and tea!" I go off to get it as she searches for her favorite afternoon show, Oprah Winfrey. Mum loves the "foo foo lah lah" of the girly communication with women, and the down to earth advice of a chap called Dr. Phil who is often featured on the show. From this time forward, if "he" is ever on the show, she will ask me to stop what I am doing and come to listen. The first time I do so to appease her, but I actually find him interesting and engaging so I continue to stop if I can whenever he comes on.

Other shows that Mum will happily watch for hours are cooking shows but I find, by and large, that they put me straight to sleep. I am happy that they fill her cup with joy, as these shows inspire her to complete her own cooking book. Not having the ability physically to write in a fluid manner any longer, she says she'll dictate the fill-in parts to me as she already has the recipes transcribed. "Lee, if I'm not able to, will you complete my recipe book for me?" she asks. "Yes, of course, Mum. It will be an honor," I assure her. I'm not sure where to start, but I'm sure I can…somehow.

The rest of the day passes quickly and then the doorbell rings, just before 6:00 p.m., signaling the curry has arrived!

Mum is quite ready. With her eyes as big as plates she anticipates a culinary delight, as dinner is something she can really look forward to. I serve it on a heated plate and on a bed tray with the trimmings and pickles, and a little glass of red wine. I arrange it and cut up her food, so she can get on with the important business of eating. With only the use of her right hand, I don't want her to have to figure what to do with large chunks of food. She is now happy, with good food, TV, home, and her own English butler. Dessert and tea finish it off, then I give her the meds.

It is now time to rest for an hour or so. I clean up and put away the leftovers. It seems like no time has passed when the doorbell rings. It is the caregiver, and time for the first trip to the little room. I announce the visitor, walk her into the room and introduce - Kate, the carer. I walk Kate around to the bathroom and show her where everything she needs is located, and how best to position the chair in the confined area. She seems quite happy with everything. I explain to Mum (in theory) what is about to happen and how. She is fine with it all.

The caregiver first empties the catheter bag. I move whatever is in the way, leave to get the wheelchair; position and lock it in place, get the lift sling and then raise the bed. Kate returns and takes the right side of the bed. I stand on the left, and together we sit Mum up, while removing all pillows. I maneuver the sling down her back, lie her gently onto the now flat bed, and then position the sling under each limb, and along her sides.

She is now secure and snug. The bed is lowered to its lowest position close to the floor. The safety bars are also lowered, and the lift is maneuvered with its legs under the bed. We lower the lift arm above the center of the patient, and each attach the sling ends to the swivel end on the lifting arm. The empty catheter bag is placed on Mum's lap.

As I slowly press the up button, the arm takes the strain. I'm constantly asking Mum if she is comfortable. As it lifts her into an upright position and takes her entire load, she mentions that the sling feels as though it is digging into her legs. It does look tight. Perhaps it's too small a sling? In the morning I will ask Julie if there is a larger sling, but for now this is all we have to work with. We swing her around as I pull the lift out from under the bed and swing it around to position her directly over the wheelchair. I push a lever with my foot and this splays the lift legs apart so that it can get closer to the wheelchair. Kate lifts the back of the sling gently as I lower Mum into the chair. We detach her sling from the lifting arm and move the lift out of the way. We each attach the chair feet and lift Mum's feet into position. She is comfortable and holding her own to sit upright. With that done, they both move out of the bedroom and to the bathroom.

While Mum and Kate are busy I shake the crumbs onto the floor, make the bed, straighten the pillows up, sweep the floor, renew her water and get ready to do the job in reverse; to situate Mum comfortably back in bed. Mean while, Kate and Mum are talking up a storm while she has a good clean up, brushes her teeth and her hair, and generally refreshes herself.

The bathroom door opens, indicating the imminent return. A joyful Mum announces she feels quite regenerated. We now begin the reverse procedure. The head pillows are positioned in an inverted V shape, so that Mum's upper back and sides and head will be well supported. With the safety bars up, I put the equipment away while Kate replaces the catheter bag and tucks Mum in. Kate rubs Mum's feet with a special deep oil to help prevent sores from developing on contact points, such as the heels. The special rolling air mattress will, we hope, take care of the rest. I put the kettle on for a lovely cup of tea, and took out some tea biscuits.

All done, Kate takes me up on my offer of tea and biscuits, and proceeds to tell Mum her entire life story. She talks...and talks. Mum inquires whether Kate will be late for her next client. She assures us that she won't and continues to talk. Twenty grueling minutes later, Mum gives me the cross-eyed look. That means:- "do something! Quickly!" I stand up and announce that it is time for her nighttime pills! They're administered, and then it's time for sleep. I offer my thanks to Kate for all she has done, as I reach out for her teacup. Kate wishes Mum a goodnight and goes off to test her next client's listening ability.

Everything has gone rather well for the first day, we both acknowledge. Mum says that after this first week of getting used to being home is over, she would like to have her friends start coming over. She also announces: "There are three things I've really wanted to happen. The first is for my final time to be at home, and I'm here; secondly, I'd like to have a tea party for my Godchildren and, finally, I'd like to have a party for as many of my friends who can come, to celebrate my life with me while I'm still here. Can you do this?" I wonder for a moment, and decide - yes, I can. I am not quite sure how or when, but I'm sure it can be done.

It is now time for bed. I make sure Mum has enough water and is otherwise warm enough and comfortable. I turn the light off, but leave the kitchen one on with the door ajar. It seems light enough, and I go back in the room to check. Mum already has her eyes closed. I sit next to her, holding her left hand, and say a prayer. Then I stroke her head for half an hour until she is fast asleep.

It is at about 02:30 a.m. that I hear the sound as I come to: "Leeeeeeeeeeeeeee!!" It is Mum calling me! I jump up, bumping into the doorway, and fall into her room thinking something is disconnected from something! Where is the emergency phone number? Or do I dial for the ambulance? But, otherwise in a complete state of shock, I quickly ask: "What is it, Mum? What's the matter!?" "Toast!" She says, "Can I have some toast and tea?" I stand in disbelief. "Are you sure, or are you dreaming, Mum?" "Oh no!" she replies, in a cheerful voice, "at the hospital, the night nurse made me toast and tea at about this time." Okay. If she wants toast and tea at two thirty in the morning, then toast and tea it is! She also wakes the TV up to see if anything is on. A short while later I carry in toast with marmalade and a nice hot cup of tea. She thanks me and asks if I can make some adjustments to her pillows and get some more water too. She then suggests I go back to bed. I don't need much persuasion, and am sound asleep in moments.

I can hear a sound as I slowly come out of my sleep. It is the alarm signaling 07:00 a.m. Time to cook breakfast! Mum is wide-awake as I pop my head into her room. "Good morning!" she says in an upbeat tone, "Can you open my curtains? I want to see what the day looks like! What's for breakfast?" She inquires. I put the kettle on and then part the curtains. I ask her, "A full breakfast?" "Oh yes please, that sounds good." Leaving out the fried bread and black pudding, I prepare a proper English breakfast which includes sizzling bacon, poached eggs, stewed tomatoes, beans on toast and toast with jam, all complemented with steaming hot tea.

I clear breakfast after it has been enjoyed and pills are given. It's 07:45 a.m. and the doorbell rings! It's Julie, with an associate, Trish, and a caregiver, Sue. Because of Sue's military-type precision and mannerisms, we soon give her the nickname: "Sergeant." I announce their arrival to Mum and she is ready. The procedure for the trip to the little room is repeated, and Sue is clearly confident and thorough. After I clean up, I have to change the sheets. The nurses help me this morning. I throw the old sheets into the washer and get it started. All else is now tidied up, it's time for some tea. Mum and "Sergeant" are still doing the morning procedures. Julie asks me about the first night. I tell her about the appetite at 02:30 a.m. and she explains the cause of that is the steroids, and asks to be advised if it continues. She produces the pill case and we put all the pills in their respective holes for the entire week. Great! I'm pleased with this little helper. It even looks less complicated just having it all together, and I'm not as likely to make a mistake.

"Sergeant" and Mum finish. We get Mum back into bed and she is ready for tea. "Sergeant" has to scoot off to her next appointment and will be back after lunch.

The nurses go in and chat with Mum, going over her condition, checking how she feels, whether all her needs are being met and whether there is any nausea or pain. They also take a few vital signs. Mum indicates all is well and that she is just glad to be home. The nurses visit the kitchen and have a quick sip of their tea. I give Mum her tea, and she turns on the TV to catch the news. Julie and Trish are happy with everything and leave to continue their day. I sit in the kitchen with my tea while the washer gives the clothes and sheets a good whirl.

By 09:30 a.m., all has quietened down from the morning rush. Mum wants to call some friends today. Arming herself with her address book and the cordless phone, she starts at it. I think, as I listen to her bubbly personality, that pretty soon she will, indeed, be ready to see friends.

It is almost ten o'clock and I ought to be thinking of lunch soon. A nice chicken salad with homemade honey mustard dressing and a small baked potato will go down well. Sounds good! If I could just get this baked potato business right and serve it before the salad goes cold... Okay, now where is that recipe book?

The washing machine reaches its final earth- shattering spin rinse, shaking everything. If I ever have to change my car engine, I'll put one of these in there and leave it on spin the cycle.

Lunch is served by twelve noon and rounded off with a small trifle and some tea. As I sit finishing my salad, Mum is glued to another one of her other favorite shows: a cooking program.

After I've seen a few blenders spin, a few chopping boards clang, and enough eggs used to warrant chickens to be a rare species, I decide these shows are only interesting for me once in a long while. Then I ponder the thought, which did come first? I am rather hoping it is the chicken, as I'm going to make a nice omelet for lunch tomorrow.

Chapter 11

"What's for dinner?"

I wash up, clear up and clean up, and then the doorbell rings. It is that time already. The Sergeant has arrived. Carefully and thoroughly Mum is spic and span and tucked back into bed in no time! The Sergeant has started to come most mornings and afternoons and has become a dear friend to Mum. We both want to salute her at times, but resist the temptation. Just as Sergeant leaves, a few minutes later "Splin" arrives. Splin is one of Mum's best friends, and a delightful person. They hug and talk, as I now go about my duties as the designated "tea boy." I do my chores, and then take advantage of their time together to go and get some shopping in and pay some bills. Splin suggests that I stop at a café and read a newspaper, and generally take my time. I'm only gone two hours, though, because I have to prepare tonight's serving of chicken baked in red wine and herbs, served with a special sauce, asparagus and small boiled potatoes. But first the order from the room is "More tea, please!" Soon after Splin leaves, promising to be back during the week with Jamaican-style cooking. Hot!

I recognize food is special to Mum, especially so at this particular time. I merely hinted at tonight's menu, and realized she now had something to look forward to. I try to make dinner, as best as I can, so that it's not just a meal but rather an *event*. I try to make the meal look just like the picture in the book, with all the garnishes, etc., and then present it with the "close-your-eyes...v-wah-lah!" type of approach. She enjoys all the extra effort so much! I serve both of us at the same time, and we're able to sit and eat together for most of the meals.

115

It doesn't seem long before the carer arrives again. After the evening routine is over, it is rest time. No more is going to happen, and we can relax for the remainder of the evening. This becomes great talk time, and Mum often wants to know how I am doing. I go on to ask her to explain how she is doing and feeling. She explains about her journey down the river and how the sense of peace is still with her. Often, when she closes her eyes, she sees the same scene: she is in the boat floating, and she feels safe and secure. "I know I am dying," she says, "I have had an amazing journey here, even though it hasn't always been the way I dreamt life would be. Yet, had anything changed, I wouldn't have experienced particular moments or met certain people that I did. Perhaps if we had had vast funds we could have done more? But you never know what lies ahead. So you are glad of what you have and what was, and is real now... right now in this very moment."

Again, we remember the good times: in India, Spain, "the Palace of Peace in London," Rome, Switzerland. There are so many places we went together and where we met so many interesting people. "Wasn't that whole time amazing?" Mum reflects, "I have visited and lived in places I never thought I would. It has, on the whole, been a wonderful life."

Out of the blue, she asks, "Lee, have I been a good Mum?" "A good Mum?" I echo, "Of course you have been a good Mum!" "For instance, do you recall when my friends used to come over to play or have dinner?" I expand. "Yes." "Well, as I told you even then, they all said at one time or another that they wished their mum could be like you. That is quite a compliment." "Yes, but how was I with the three of you kids and your father?"

"Hmmmmm…well, for what you had to deal with and the tools that were available to you during that time, you did a lot. You did the best you could do, Mum, and that is all anyone can expect of anyone. We had three meals a day, clothes, and a roof over our heads. We all grew up knowing right from wrong, to be kind and thoughtful of others, to treat people as we wanted to be treated, to be selfless, to help others, to be truthful, honest and strong, and not afraid. I haven't always got it right myself, but I'm working on it. Mum, we had the best meals! I am not afraid to try any food, if only once. We had the best bedtime stories, magic dust, comfort, love, laughs and hugs. There are so many ways to acknowledge that you have been a good mum, but you've heard most of them all before. Most important of all, you loved us."

With that, shedding a tear, she demands a hug, asks for more tea and wonders what we have for snacks and whether there is any ice cream…

Her left arm is quite cold. She says it doesn't seem to get warm; it is as if it is cold to the bone. I massage the arm from shoulder to fingertips, until she can feel it is warm and relaxes enough to sleep. I pray over her and kiss her goodnight. I have developed a light-sleeping mode and I can sleep listening, "with one ear open."

A big clang and a few words of frustration wake me up this early morning. As I get to the room, I discover the floor is wet. Mum has accidentally knocked a plastic water bottle off the table because she has had difficulty reaching it. I fashion a small holding basket out of a coat hanger, loose enough for the bottle to fit in, and position and secure it in an easier-to-reach place. It works well and she is pleased. "Could you make me some tea while you're up," she enquires. "Of course... any toast with that?" I ask, and then am soon back in bed and fast asleep.

Jasmine calls, as she often does, with a great idea. Although she isn't able to be there to help directly, she can cook and freeze a load of food for Mum, and on nights or days that I'm too tired to cook I can take a meal out of the freezer in the morning and heat it up in the microwave at lunchtime or at night. She and Mike come over the following weekend and fill up the freezer with frozen chili and bolognaise sauce. I am truly grateful. They stay for most of the day, allowing me to go into town and do some shopping and to sit and have tea out, some place away from the "Goldfish Bowl."

I can tell that after these last two months with Mum at home, I am already feeling tired. Mum is getting a little irritable at times. She is lying there day after day with no hope and one ultimate destiny (which is true for us all, but we usually don't have to face it in this manner). It's stressful! The stress of being in one spot, with no real hope of improving, is getting to her and there isn't much opportunity to change that perspective in any significant way.

The following morning is bright and sunny. Spring is truly in the air. Mum seems quite cheery this morning. Enthused by the sun and the many happy thoughts of warm English summers, she says "I would love to see the garden." "How about sitting in the wheel chair today so that I can take you to your garden for a little while? Do you feel strong enough?" I ask. She hesitates for a moment, smiles and says, "Yeahhhh! Okay, let's go!" After she completes her morning activities, we assist her back to her room where she is initially raised off the chair. A section is put in and a special sponge cushion is placed on top before we lower her back down. We cover her in blankets and otherwise make her comfortable. She smiles and is excited about this simple opportunity to go outside once more to her beloved garden area.

We make our way past the passage to the bathroom. Amy the carer is in front; I am behind. Amy stops to open the front door. The bottom of the front door has an overhang with a draft excluder hanging down from it, sort of like a short brush running along the width of the door. The passage is narrow at this point, so one has to get the right side wheels to go on the sturdy overhanging part, and lift the others off the floor two inches, to level Mum's ride till she is out of the door and all the wheels come to rest. She pays no attention to all the lifting, heaving and puffing that is required to get her outside. Mum is beaming with a smile from ear to ear. How pleased she is just to be here, outside in the sun! We position her in a nice sunny spot next to her clean wooden potting table and lock the wheels.

Amy has to leave, although she will be back after lunch. I return inside to get a cup of tea, then I sit with mine on the steps in front of Mum, having placed hers on the table.

She listens to a blackbird warbling its tune and watches it hop on the tree branches and then to the garden. She studies the grass, looking at the general shape of the garden, and what is in her plant pots. She points out a tall plant growing significantly out of a pot, and explains that it started as a big pip from an avocado fruit she once had with her salad. "I kept the pip in water till it sprouted a long root, and then I planted it. Three years later, here it is!" It is now about three feet tall with large shiny green leaves.

Mum sips her tea, enjoying every morsel of this moment. She feels led to remind me that each moment is a precious one, and that now is the only time we really have. It is interesting how we so often look ahead to our destination in life instead of enjoying the journey, we muse. It is a reflection of life in the modern world-the "normal" pressures of everyday life with places to go, people to see, things to do and deals to be made. These often cause us to forget simply to stop to smell the roses, or to spend time with those near and dear to us. Time is the most precious commodity we have. Yet we give it away so freely without a thought, and it is gone once the moment has passed. "Use your moments and spend them wisely," a wise man once told me. We often enjoy sharing such ponderous reflections about life.

Mum sheds some tears as we sit there, enjoying… now. She is so happy to be outside, and has missed the freedom to be able to come here. She reminds me again of the two other things she wants to do, now that she is home: one is to have a tea party with her Godchildren, those of Splin and her sisters, the other - a last party with her dearest friends. "I will see how I can get those things moving and will let you know when I do," I promise. Forty-five minutes later sitting upright is looking a little uncomfortable. Mum acknowledges that she is feeling a bit tired and would like to lie down on her bed. So back into the house we go. I realize that it is just me helping her now. I say nothing and manage to get her back in to the house without too much effort. I position her as we have been positioning her together, attaching all the sling ends of the mechanical octopus, and slowly lift her up. A few moments later she is relaxing, snug as a bug in bed.

She wants to sleep for a while, so I close her curtains and the doors returning to the kitchen. I finish clearing and cleaning, and begin to write down ideas, names and numbers for the parties.

One of Mum's dear friends, Natasha, who comes over now and again, stops by this morning while Mum is sleeping. I quietly tell her about both the parties. She is most interested in helping with the Godchildren's party, having a child of her own and being used to arranging children's parties, and will get back to me with some ideas during the week.

Mum calls. She is waking up and wants a hot drink - coffee, made with hot milk. She enjoys this as a treat from time to time. I mention that Natasha is helping me put some ideas together for her Godchildren's party, and that I'll plan her friends' party next.

Mum asks, "Will you ring my sisters, Monique, in Spain and, Katherine, in the South of France? Your Auntie Marion gave me their numbers when we last spoke, and I've been wondering when to call them. It has been so long, so many years, since we have said hello. How do I call to say goodbye? Will you call first?" "Of course I will," I reply.

I can hear the phone ring in Spain. It makes a different ringing sound. A soft woman's voice, speaking Spanish, comes on the line. I explain who I am and there is silence for a moment. "Lee, oh my word! How are you? I haven't seen you since you were a little boy! Where are you calling from? What are you doing? How is Baby?" We quickly get to the Baby part, then, and after I explain her present situation again there is silence on the other end. I ask whether this is a good moment. She says, "Give me your number and I'll call back shortly." We chat a while longer and then hang up. I call the number in Nice in France. There is no answering machine and no answer from Katherine. I'll try again later.

The sun still shines outside Mum's room and it is a genuinely nice day for a change. The phone rings. Mum has the cordless handset on her bed and answers the call. From her gasp and surprise, I know it is her younger sister, Monique. It is hard to imagine even a condensed version of twenty-years of catch-up talk between sisters. They have a good try, anyhow. I leave the room until Mum calls me a while later, asking for more tissues. I'm sure Monique has a box at her end too. I leave the room again, retreating to the "fish bowl." I make a beef strip organic salad with a light balsamic vinegar dressing for lunch today.

I hear laughter, chatter, silence and then more laughter coming from Mum's room. It is almost an hour and a half later when she calls me. She has hung up the phone and looks happy, but sad. I comfort her and congratulate her for making the effort to connect with her sisters. Through her tears, she says, "I can't remember why the silence between us was so long. Please stay in touch with your aunts and cousins after all this, won't you?" "Yes," I agree, "I will."

"How about a nice salad, Mum? It's lunchtime." "Okay! And what's for dessert?" "Errr... ice cream & fresh strawberries." It isn't long before the usual time arrives and the little trip is underway. Today has seemed like a long day already, and it is barely half through. Mum is back in bed, noticeably tired. This is possibly also due to the emotional drain of her chat earlier and her thoughts since.

I ponder dinner preparations. I've planned something special for tonight. Dinner will be white fish, slowly cooked inside a blanket of pastry, with a rich white wine sauce poured over it at serving time. Baby carrots and sweet peas will accompany the meal and a small glass of wine, and crème brulèe for dessert, will top it all off. She'll like this, I'm sure. Mum watches Oprah and cooking shows until dinnertime.

I sit and think about these last few months and my routine at this point. It proceeds as follows. I am up at around 06:30 / 07:00 a.m. to make breakfast, give medications and make tea. At 08:00 a.m., I assist the care nurses, make tea, change sheets, get the washing machine going, clear up, make more tea, change music, make MORE tea and answer the phone. At 11:00 a.m. I prepare lunch, give medications, make yet more tea and assist the care nurses. At 1:30 p.m., I again make tea, admit more guests, hang up the washing around the flat and over the doors, do shopping, do the banking, take care of bills, go to corner shop, make tea again, of course, and serve more guests. By 5:00 p.m., it is time to prepare dinner, give medications and assist the care nurses. At 7:30 p.m., I clean up and make another round of tea. At 9:30 p.m., I give night meds, make nighttime drinks and sandwiches, watch some TV with Mum, hug her, tuck her in for the night, pray with her, kiss her goodnight, and then at 11:00 p.m., finally, it is "Lee time" - to read or just collapse! It always seems to go pretty much this way day in, day out. I'm fine doing this as long as it needs to be done. The rest of life can wait!

It is dinnertime, and the meal is a hit with Mum. During dinner, she reflects on her conversation with Aunt Monique. She and her husband of almost thirty-five years, Martin, have retired from their business in Brussels, Belgium, and bought a place on the coast in Spain. It is, apparently, in a nice location away from popular tourist areas. Of their three children, all boys, one is married living in Switzerland, one works in South America and the other in Brussels. Monique, too, doesn't have a really close relationship with any of the other sisters, except for Katherine in France. She and Mum both expressed regrets concerning each others' absence for so many years of their lives and, regardless of the circumstances (as sad as they are), they agreed it was still good to talk. They plan to do this regularly from now on. Monique will call again in a few days and will talk with Katherine in the meantime as well.

It has been a nice day, and after the evening's routines are over Mum wants to go to sleep a little earlier than usual.

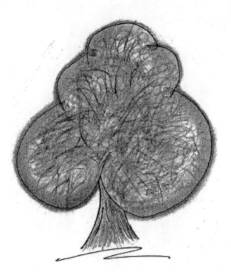

Chapter 12

Gifts of love through words and a beautiful broach

A pile of post arrived today, along with at least six cards for Mum from the U.S. We open them after the morning's routine is done. With a beaker of fresh tea, Mum reads the cards. I don't recognize the addresses and notice they are from different cities across America. Oddly each one has a picture of a bird. They are the sweetest encouragement cards sent together, with poems, prayers and love. Mum is very touched by their words and sentiment. I soon find out that Joel in Tampa contacted Christians via the internet, explained the predicament and said nothing more. Over the next few months, one hundred and eighty six cards come through the door. I hang them on string from one side of the wall to the other in Mums view, on graduated levels, and then do the same behind her bed as there are so many. Each card is a gift of love from a well-wishing person who took a little time to pick a card, write in a prayer or a few carefully chosen words, and then mailed it.

Some time ago, soon after Mum arrived home, during one brief conversation with Joel, he had asked what Mum loves to see. After we got through a few different thoughts, I said birds! She loves to see and hear birds. I had heard and thought nothing more about his question until the cards started to come in. They all had different types of birds on them.

One pastor and his wife from Nebraska, U.S., sent the most exquisitely colored broach, in the form of a peacock, from their personal collection. In an accompanying note, he told Mum that he and his wife had anointed the broach with oil and prayed over it. Mum was so touched by their kindness and thoughtfulness; it truly strengthened her spirits for a long while. "Perhaps I'll be able to say "thank you" in person when I get back?" I wonder.

Many friends and neighbors come and go. The neighbors come mostly in the evenings and are very considerate, both with their time and of Mum's ability to have only light conversation. They often bring fresh flowers. Many friends and members of groups she belongs to also come during the day, and others call on the phone. It gets to a point where Mum is a little overwhelmed, and she explains how some people tell her all of their problems. She listens without really wanting to know more, but out of loving concern begins to become burdened with other people's baggage. She feels she is trying to let go of her own at this time, not to take on more. One totally inconsiderate person tries to sell her a cancer cure over the phone.

I take a fairly strong approach to this growing concern, and post a note on the front and back doors which briefly encourages everybody to leave *any* personal problems outside, and NOT to bring them in to discuss or explain to Mum. I overhear one man going on about his doomed relationship and I decide to intervene gently. I explain Mum's predicament, he says he understands and nothing more needs to be said. The doctor likes the idea of the notes and comments and points out that oddly enough people are often inclined to discuss their own problems at such times.

128

I am doing okay, but feeling markedly tired. Natasha comes to the door and suggests that as she has a few hours to spare, I could take off for a while and go for a walk. We chat first about the Godchildren's party date, agree times and plan what we hope will occur. Great!

As Mum and Natasha get on with serious girl talk I step outside, while the clouds gather, just in time for them to let rip with torrential rain as I reach the end of the street. My thought is to head directly to the indoor shopping center, determined to take a walk and have a little break. So I do. I take three hours and am glad of the time out. On the way home, I stop at a fish and chip shop. I order two cod and chips, plus some pickled onions, which will make a nice treat. I arrive back just in time for Natasha to leave to pick up her daughter from the nursery round the corner.

In the morning, the DN Julie arrives. The first thing she says is, "Lee, you look tired! Do you know that we have a system whereby we can have a nurse come and sit in with your mum (say - one evening a week) and you can go out to have a meal, or go and see a film and just relax? We also ought to think, perhaps, of having your mum go to a weekend care center. She could actually go for up to five days. Believe it or not, that would give her a break as well as you. You could stay there, too; there are lots of staff and volunteers. They specialize in terminally ill patients. I'll mention it to your mum when we talk, but we need to start organizing a night off for you at least once a week, as soon as possible, before you collapse." I have been doing my best and although I want to be Superman, I realize I'm only human. I am indeed getting tired but am still functioning well, although I don't quite know how.

Perhaps in such situations we draw on energy reserves we didn't even know we have? Grace is the only thing I can put it down to - the invisible but constant help and support I am reminded of continually through 'coincidences,' (or Godcidences) apparently random encounters, a sudden access of strength when I've been flagging, and so on. I wonder how people cope in such situations when they have no faith in a higher power or an order somewhere above and beyond the chaos. That must be truly hard.

It is mid afternoon when Aunt Monique from Spain phones. We chat briefly before I hand her over to Mum. They talk for a good hour, and then Mum says: "Here! Monique wants a word with you..." We have a quick chat and she says she is proud of me for what I am doing for Mum. She proceeds to throw me completely by suggesting that, if possible, I should consider letting Mum have some pot! She has a friend who went through a similar situation and it really calmed him down and eased the pain and stress when he had some. He didn't smoke, so he had it in some little cakes. I acknowledge what my aunt is saying, but feel clueless in this area. It just so happens that Mum has recently been hinting that she'd like to be able to smoke a simple rollup, not a cigarette from a pack. I am not sure what to say, but I thank Monique for the thought. She also mentions that she may consider flying over, or perhaps I can fly over there before I leave to return to the U.S.? We say our goodbyes and she tells me she will call again.

As the next week passes by, it is apparent that Mum is becoming increasingly frustrated. She doesn't seem to be able to focus her attention and can't read for long anymore. Most significantly, her memory and concentration are being affected and she tires more easily. Her appetite hasn't changed, though.

I get a call from the relief organization. It provides qualified nurses who will even relieve me from cooking on those particular nights. The lady indicates that Friday nights will be available for me to take off from 6:30 p.m. till 11:30 p.m., which sounds like enough time for a dinner and a movie to me! Sure, okay...let's arrange it.

Mum is fine with this proposal; indeed, she is glad that I will have the chance to relax a bit. The week passes by and Friday night arrives. I make dinner so that all the nurse has to do is serve it. When she arrives, I say "See you later!" and leave by 6:40 p.m.

The mall is my first thought, to choose one of the many restaurants in which to eat. It is a little quiet when I arrive and, as I look around, I realize that all the shops are closing... at 7:00 p.m.! Outside, the other eating establishments in the vicinity closed by 5:30 p.m. This, of course, is England! In the U.S., most things are open till at least 11:00 p.m. and many twenty four hours. I'll check out the movie times and then find a nearby pub! I am thinking of the AMC 24, and other such large U.S. establishments. I find the local Odeon 3. Wow! All of three movies to choose between! The next one starts at 8:30 p.m., so I'll need to be back by 8:15 p.m. In the meantime, I'll check out a pub for food.

I find one quite close by, and wade through the smoke to find a table near a door. I put my jacket down, pick up a menu and go to place my order. The room is full of people all ready for a fun weekend, and this place is as good as any to start off, I guess. Groups of people and friends are chatting, laughing and enjoying the moment, their upbeat spirits helped along by beer and wine. Standing at the counter I put in an order for some hot food, opting for the pub special; fresh "shepherd's pie" (Which will undoubtedly be a wonderful frozen creation they will microwave just for me!)

131

I also order lemonade and lime with ice and a hot coffee for after dinner. They look at me suspiciously... we don't have ice.

I sit for a few moments, looking around and listening to the constant but unclear chatter, when I suddenly feel alone among the crowd-just me, myself and I. The door opens as a few more people enter and I gulp in some fresh air before it closes again. To my great relief, I find part of a newspaper - at least I can avert my eyes from people, now that I am already bored with counting the pictures on the wall, wondering how many words I can make out of "Exit" and reading the ingredients on the back of the tomato sauce bottle.

I quickly turn the pages looking for an interesting article, and there it is...four pages of nothing but stock quotes! The meal arrives with my cold drink and coffee. I thank the waitress and wait another minute. Apparently you have to eat with your fingers, so I get up to go and find some silverware and anything else I might need. Service and this pub are two concepts that don't go together. The phone rings. "Hi, Mum!" "Lee, where are you?" "Mum, I'm out having a wonderful meal. Why? What's the matter?" I ask. "Oh, nothing... What time will you be back?" "By about 11:30 p.m." "Could you come back sooner?" She inquired. "Well, if the movie finishes sooner I will." "Okay then. Bye Lee." "Okay, 'bye Mum." I leave soon after I finish my cold coffee, and am in plenty of time for the movie. I turn the phone on to "vibrate."

At last, time to sit back and simply relax... The phone vibrator goes off. I leave my seat. "Mum, are you alright?" "Yes." "As soon as the movie is over I'll be right back. Are you sure you're okay mum?" "Yeah." "Okay then. Bye-bye." After another hour so the phones goes off for the third time. I leave my seat and suggest: "Mum, give me a yes or no…are you free to talk?" "No." "Is the carer in the room?" "Yes." "Is she treating you okay?" "Yes." "Is she doing something that is driving you bonkers?" "Yes." "Okay then…errr… is she talking incessantly?" "Yes." "Is everything else otherwise okay?" "Yes." "I'll be home soon, Mum. Okay?" "Okay then. Bye Lee."

I decide that I'm going to have to come to another arrangement, although the idea of time off is a nice thought. I'll call DN Julie and see what we can do. I go back in to try to catch the end of the film just as everyone starts to get up and leave, so I head home as quickly as possible.

After next morning's breakfast and morning routine is over, I go in to Mum with a cup of tea. She says, "Lee, I want to have a smoke!" Having had lung cancer, I wonder whether she will be okay if she does so. When I ask her whether she thinks she will be affected because of the previous lung cancer, she embarks upon what I can only describe as an immediate "food and communication strike." I try to reason with her but she refuses to talk, apart from mumbles and telling me to go away.

I call her doctor for advice. He is quite calm, first of all reminding me that, when Mum gets upset, it is because of her predicament and is not meant, or directed at me, personally. I explain the whole situation. The doctor indicates that indeed smoking is likely to cause her to cough, that she might experience some discomfort and that, under normal circumstances, this should not be permitted. However, at this stage in my mum's situation, without going over the top - I can let her have a few hand rolled cigarettes a day or anything else she wants, within reason. I thank the doctor for his thoughts and for being down-to-earth. Mum also has cravings for chocolate, cake and other sweets. I know that, because of her diabetes, her sugar levels have to be monitored to make sure she doesn't go into a comatose state. The doctor says he will set up some additional medication to overcome high sugar levels. As soon it is arranged, we'll let her have whatever she wants and monitor her on a daily basis, administering medication as needed.

I leave via the back door, walk to the Indian corner shop and bring back some loose tobacco and some roll-up papers. I sit back in the "goldfish bowl," trying to learn how to roll cigarettes. The first three are a disaster… so are the next two. The sixth one looks like a roll-up cigarette, though a bit soggy.

I make an ashtray out of tin foil, and armed with the roll-up and a lighter, I open Mum's door, quickly announcing the all-clear to have a smoke! She doesn't budge. She is still too upset. I leave the roll-up for her on her table and back out into the kitchen. It is a strange moment. My question to her was one of care, concern and love. I actually had not told her "no." It is the fact that she cannot just choose for herself that frustrates her to this point. She continues in this frame of mind right through lunchtime, refusing to eat. That time has arrived and Mum doesn't care to be moved or bothered. I take Amy into the kitchen and explain everything so that she can understand basically what initiated this dramatic change in mood. Amy goes into the room and chats with Mum, who reiterates her desire to stay put. So Amy just tidies up around her, rubbing her feet and arm, and tucking the blankets in…and that is that.

Amy explains that she has seen this type of mood swing on a number of occasions and, before she leaves, assures me that Mum will be her usual self again soon. It seems best to just let her be... until she wants otherwise. If Mum needs to take a trip sooner rather than later then call our number and another carer will come out as soon as it's possible. Okay thanks, I will. She leaves. I sit back in the kitchen and decide to make some more roll-ups while I have the time. I need the practice, anyway.

I hour or so later, I can hear Mum mumbling and getting aggravated, so I ask if she needs help. "I can't get this silly lighter to work," she says. I find another in the drawer and light it as she puts the roll-up to her lips. She draws in a deep breath as the end of the roll up glows brightly. She immediately coughs and sputters as she blows out a gray cloud of smelly smoke. "Oh that was good! Thanks, Lee," as she coughs and puffs some more. I quickly leave the room. I'm not able to be around cigarette smoke. The smell simply turns my stomach.

The call for tea soon comes. I bring in a fresh cup and Mum apologizes, "I'm sorry for being such a pain!" I give her a hug and tell her that under the circumstances, she has been really great. While she drinks her tea, I tell her the gist of the conversation with the doctor, with which she is pleased. Then she adds, "This is all the time I have, and the worst that can happen with these roll-ups is that I'll die. We already know that it is going to happen anyway. I don't want to have to worry about smoking or what I eat anymore. I may have five minutes, five days, or a few more months, but I want to enjoy what I can at this point." "I understand exactly where you are coming from, and I'll do my best to help you do just that," I reply, just glad we are back to "normal" again.

Chapter 13

"The egg has been laid!"

"When is Amy coming back?...because I need to take a quick trip," comes the urgent question from Mum's room. "Well, hang on...I have to call the company and then they will send someone over." "You'd better call them quick!" I do, and there is no answer, so I leave a message. Mum asks again when will they come. "Errr... well, there isn't anyone there and I just left a message." "I can't wait! I need to go!" "Well, ummm... errrr, I can handle getting you in the little room." "Okay then, but you'd get me there fast!"

I position the equipment. I find it difficult to roll her back and forth into the sling and work the lift alone, but I manage and get her situated into the wheelchair. "You'd better hurry!" "Okay Mum... hold on! No accidents on the way!" I say, as I maneuver her down the passage, to the little room, and into her final position. Locking the wheels, I leave her and go to straighten her bed. I am pleased with myself that nothing happened on the way and that I did this by myself. Fifteen minutes later I hear, "Okay, I'm done!" As I go to maneuver her out, she says, "Oh wait. You need to cleanse me with the baby wipes! With rapid instructions she says, "position the wheelchair over there; the gloves the nurse uses are behind, and the bowl is here. You'll need to flush the wipes and then rinse the bowl and dispose of everything else in the plastic bag. Then you can wash my face and take me back."

I freeze, for a milli-second, wondering what to do! I once helped out some friends by baby-sitting for them. I'd hoped the baby would hold out till the parents returned, but she didn't. By the time I had finished, I had the stuff on my arms, the baby's legs and on the changing table. We got it worked out eventually though, and the baby giggled throughout.

I quickly come to the conclusion, concerning the current situation, that this is what it must be like to be a parent, and that this is how Mum took care of us as children. So this is like a role reversal... I can do this, if she could have done that. I don the gloves, doing just as she has said. I am done in just a few minutes, and add, "Good girl! You did a great job!" And that is that. I have her all tucked back in bed a short while later, and ready for something to eat.

Her discomfort and intenseness increases over the next week. It is at this time that Mum says, "Lee, I called a friend who contacted a friend of a friend. You need to take twenty pounds, put it in a jam jar with a lid and leave it behind the white flowerpot under the potting table." "What am I doing this for?" "Well, there will be some special roll-ups there for me between this afternoon and 9:00 p.m." "How special are these roll-ups?" "They will help me relax and sleep better. You can't imagine the stress I feel just lying here." "You mean, 'Smokey Joe?'" "Yes." She said. "I understand. It's okay, Mum, I understand." "Thank you for understanding."

I walk outside and feel very guilty somehow for what I am now doing. Consequently, I pretend to arrange the flowers and the pots, and admire the garden. I walk about as if I actually have a clue about gardening. I return to the pots to make a final adjustment and slide the jam jar behind the white flowerpot.

I stand up, glancing once more at the wonderful garden that I have had very little to do with creating. I think for a second a satellite is probably watching me at this very moment and teams of armed men in black outfits are following my every move, waiting for the signal to burst through the doors and windows, hanging from helicopters! Or maybe I've seen too many films???

Walking back into the flat, I'm feeling quite uneasy. "THE EGG HAS BEEN LAID!" I say out loud. [Perhaps they'll wait until I return at 9:00 p.m.? I dread the thought of returning.] "You what?" Mum asks. "The EGG is positioned for the eagle. The egg has been laid. I put the you-know-what by the flowerpot. Mum, I'm using code lingo here!"

The rest of the afternoon goes by and, at about 4:00 p.m., Mum's friend Francis stops over to give her a massage on her left arm and side. "More tea, please!" The evening comes, Francis leaves, and dinner is served. I retreat to the kitchen and close the door as Mum enjoys a roll-up soon after dinner. She watches the T.V. I sit listening for the helicopters. The carer comes to assist with Mum's needs. It is much easier doing this with two, but I know now that if the worst comes to the worst, I can handle it alone. The carer leaves after all is complete, and more tea is put on.

It has seemed like an eternity but then, before you can say, "Can't we put this off and figure out something else?" It is nine o'clock. Perhaps Mum has forgotten ?... Just then, a loud voice comes from the room, "Lee, it's nine o'clock! Go and see!" "Yes, yes, I know! I'll be back in a sec." I open the front door and can't hear any helicopters. All is quiet. [Perhaps... too quiet? Is this the calm before the storm – troopers?] I grab the broom and decide

139

to sweep around the area, just so that I can glance around and see if anyone is watching, or looking suspicious or out of the ordinary (Wait! I'm sweeping the garden at 9:00 p.m...). I expertly drop the broom by the potting table and bend down to grab it. Swooping up the jam jar, I place it into my jacket pocket at the same time. I stand up to admire the sweeping job, the result of which I can hardly see because it is dark, and then I walk back inside.

I realize that I'm shaking. I make sure the curtains are closed in the kitchen before taking the jar out of my pocket. Inside, I count fifteen fat roll-ups with pointy ends in a plastic bag! I call out, "Mum, THE EAGLE HAS LANDED!" "The what did what???" I repeat myself, more softly this time, "The-Eagle-Has-Landed!" "What on earth are you talking about??" "Mum... I'm still using the code...you know... the egg, the eagle! The package has been dropped. The goodies are in the bag! You know, the jam jar, Smokey Joes!" "Ohhh...they're here? Well, why didn't you just say so? Okay, bring me one, then!" The thought crosses my mind that my father would be proud of me about now.

Opening the plastic bag, I pull one out and hand it over. She inspects it, smells it and then lights it. The end lights up and then glows red. When she exhales, the smell is nauseating! I leave the room quickly and she apologizes. I tell her not to worry about it as I close the door. I hope this smelly stuff helps her pain and frame of mind.

I sit in the "goldfish bowl" and think that this little space in the kitchen will probably become more my home than ever as the smoking and Joes continue from here on. I think about turning on the big fan and opening the front window so that her room doesn't smell like an old ashtray. Tomorrow morning I'll work out a system to rid her room of the smell of stale smoke. I proceed quickly to make sure that my bedroom door is closed and the passage door from the front room is too, so that the flat in general doesn't smell either. I can hear her cough and sputter. "Are you alright in there?" I enquire. "Oh yeah, I'm fine…(cough, cough.)"

I catch up with some writing and put a few thoughts on paper. I often play upbeat contemporary Christian music, as I find it comforting and uplifting during times when I feel tired and weary. I seem to feel this way more and more of late. I think of the many people around the world who right now are doing the same as I am, and more, for loved ones and I wonder how they, too, cope with all this.

Soon comes the inevitable tea order! I open the door and the air is thick. I have to put the fan on just to try to clear the air. I give Mum her tea and biscuits. "How are you feeling now, Mum?" "I feel…better, mellow, relaxed. In fact, the tightness in my head has gone. I feel good. How amazing is that? I think I will sleep well tonight. I'm sorry that you have to leave. I know you can't stand the smell of cigarettes." "Not a problem, Mum. You don't need to worry. You just need to feel the best you can." This does help Mum for a little while. It clearly takes the edge off of her stress and pain.

There is much chatter with Splin since the party for her children, Mum's Godchildren, is to be this weekend. Natasha has arranged for a puppeteer to provide entertainment and has taken care of the catering.

Sunday afternoon arrives, and Mum is excited to see the kids. There are eight children, and a couple of adults present. It is such a fun day for them and Mum. The puppeteer sets up in Mum's room to her right, three feet from the end of her bed, and the kids sit carefully on her left as he prepares to begin a pirate show, in which they are all to be participants. He gives Mum a part, for which she does great and is right on cue. We all really enjoy ourselves. It is an animated pirate story in which the "baddies" lose and the "goodies" win. Everybody sings and laughs and has such a good time. The kids then leave the room and all have lunch on Mum's grass lawn in the sun. There are…can you guess???… tea, drinks, sandwiches and cake for all, and then there are gifts for each child.

After the singer is all sung out, and the kids have played enough to be worn out, it is time for home. They all line up and each enters the room to hug Mum. She lowers the bed to be more at their level, and they all say "thank you" and "I love you." Mum thanks them and tells them she loves them, too. It is a sweet time, even though they don't understand her tears. It is to be the last time she will see them on earth. They all go home happily, full of cake, tea, joy and love.

I video the event from start to finish, and Mum enjoys reliving it after the event. The day was as wonderful as everyone had hoped it might be.

Mum sleeps well this night, feeling almost fulfilled in her final wishes. There will be one last party with her friends. But for now, it is time to sleep. "Sleep well, Mum," I kiss her head and leave her sleeping in peace.

The morning comes and Mum has a light breakfast. She is quite peaceful on this day. No 'Joes'... just staring out of the window. She says that last night she felt, and this morning woke up with, the same peace she has been feeling, and the sense of that journey on the river is still with her. "If I close my eyes, I can still feel the warmth of Him gently stroking my shoulder and my head." She beams a contented smile and I can feel her peace. I, too, can relax immediately this morning. There is a peace spoken of in the Bible that is "beyond all understanding." I conclude that this must be what we are experiencing.

Today I'll use up some more of Jasmine's delightful bolognaise dish which Mum really likes. I'll let Mum continue to rest. I decide to write a poem from Mum's perspective, as I imagine it, for the nurses and carers while I have the opportunity.

Oh, what a day it has been!

What a day it has been!
People have won medals;
battles have been fought...
There has been happiness and tragedies all over.
Much has happened and many a foot has tread
- I've heard it and seen it all,
right from my bed.

The Angels they come so far
with their concerns about me;
Each day they show up to care,
with the tons of love that they share.
How long has it been now?
How much longer will it be?
Oh what a day it has been!

I see people walk by my window with cheer.
I watch on, with my tea and smokes at hand.
Oh Lee, roll me another, my dear.
Friends and well wishers come in
with thoughts and hidden fears.
I tell them it's all right,
there is no fear here.
I think I'll take a nap.

Is it dinner already?
Why am I feeling so hungry?
A curry would be nice-
I hope I get loads of rice!
I'll try to get more in my belly
and less on the sheet.
Oh, and my favorite show just came on the telly.

Well the day is over, as I lie here and wonder
will I wake up in Bristol or in the warmth of eternal light?
I'll just sleep on it for now,
feeling always grateful for yet another day that I've seen.
How precious life is and
what another wonderful day it has been!

~ ✦ ~

Chapter 14

She's celebrating her life, too.

The following week, the final preparations for Mum's party are made and Saturday will be the day. I ask those who live locally to bring a dish of something. I'll make a special and delicious Malaysian dish called "Tomato Breedy," and will supply the sodas, dips, crisps and nuts. I've opted for paper plates, cups, and other disposable items, so that I won't create a washing up mountain. As people are coming from a distance, too, there will be no set time and it will all have to work around Mum's regular daily routine with nurses and carers. I imagine people will begin arriving from the afternoon onwards and stay until...well, until it makes sense to leave. We certainly and collectively want Mum to absorb all the love and goodness she can from all of her friends. It will be another special day.

Saturday arrives and Mum is all excited. Splin came early to do her hair and all the "foo-foo-lah-lah" girlie stuff. She has on her best nightdress, has fresh sheets and covers, and is nearly ready to hit the town. I have cooked a huge pot of the Malaysian dish last night and now I just need to do the rice. I get it started, and then put out the other snack foods and condiments.

Two of Mum's treasured friends, Michelle and Cynthia, from London arrive first. They stopped off on the way over to pick up a few things. There are many kisses, hugs and greetings as friends meet. I put on the tea. Next come Marianne and her daughter, Savannah, from Exeter in Southern England, two bright and cheerful souls. It is already like a girls' school reunion.

145

I just let them all get on with it and, like every good "tea boy," keep the hot beverage flowing. Michael and Sam arrive, then Adrian & Laura and Mum's dear neighbors and other friends. From that point on the place just fills up and spills out onto the back lane. A large group stays in the kitchen where the music is playing. The drinks are flowing. The air is alive with chatter and laughter. As Mum can handle them, a couple of people visit two at a time and close the door behind them. They chat and hug; much joy emanates from her room. As they come back out, others enter, it's non-stop. Soon it is dinnertime and Mum needs a few moments alone, just to eat and rest. The carer arrives after this, and all is taken care of in short order so as to accommodate Mum's visitors. Once the coast is all clear, more friends take time to visit with Mum. Most people know each other; those who don't soon get acquainted.

They nearly all have a story about how Mum has touched their lives in some special way. Her sisters aren't able to come and Jasmine doesn't like crowds: They are missed. Mum feels loved and cared for, and is clearly touched by her friends being here. It is good to see her joy.

I am having a tough time pushing the Tomato Breedy today. I keep announcing, "Big demand for Tomato Breedy! Another batch is on its way!" and "There is another run on the Tomato Breedy! Quick! Take some now while you still can!" Followed by, "Please, everyone, wait your turn; women and children first; don't push! Let those who haven't had some ... have some! Errr... it's FREE! Okay, I'll pay you! Ello??? Anyone???"

At this rate I am going to be eating this wonderful Malaysian dish three times a day for the next two weeks.

Mum calls to me, and by the look in her eyes I can discern that she is tired and needs to rest a while. What tires her most is trying to concentrate on what is being said by someone and trying to take it in, understand and then reply. Her ability to do this is becoming quite stretched, and she can't focus well. But she knows clearly who everyone is, and is so happy they have all come to see her. Mum is becoming more tired as the weeks are going by. Today's look is tired but happy, with an air of complete contentedness. This is just what she has wanted. What a *privilege* it is to be a part of this special day for her!

~ ✣ ~

The Saturday Carer

I get a new offer of time off. Now it will be Saturdays I get a break, as the administrators have introduced a new carer who is able to be here all day until the early evening. I feel I can do more during the day on Saturday than I can on a Friday night. A week later, I meet the carer a little after all the morning's procedures. A pleasant, rotund lady who has never missed a meal, she has brought with her reading material, which is good as I have to explain that she can only go into the room to check on Mum, or if Mum calls her. Otherwise it is important to leave her alone.

I organize Mum's dinner in advance on this first Saturday, so that when I get back I won't have anything to do. Indeed, Mum is looking forward to Cornish pasty (a tasty meat and vegetable pie) this evening. I ask the carer to put the oven on at 5:30 p.m. so that dinner will be ready for Mum when I get in at 6:00 p.m. I have a good day walking around the city seeing the sights and going down by the waterside. The exercise is welcome, and I return feeling refreshed at by the evening time.

I walk in right at 6:00 p.m. The carer is waiting with her coat on, eager to go, as she has to catch a bus. I thank her and she scoots off at a purposeful pace. The smell of freshly cooked pastry is wafting through the air. I wash my hands, get the tray ready, open the still-warm oven and...no pasty?! I look in the fridge...not there. I look and can see pastry flakes on the counter. I look in the sink and there is a plate with pastry flakes, ketchup and a residue of mashed potato and peas. I call out, dreading the answer, "Mum, have you already had dinner?" "No, not yet." "Well we have been struck by the notorious pasty eater!" I announce. "You mean she ate my dinner?" Mum inquires pitifully. "I'm sorry to say that indeed she has! I think she thought I meant the dinner was for her, and eat by six before I get back?" "Lee, you know what I fancy then? Steak and kidney pie and small chips!"

I dash out for just five minutes around the corner to the take-away, and Mum is soon enjoying her pie. That carer becomes known as the "pasty eater" and I make extra food available for the next time she is on duty.

~ ✦ ~

More chocolates please

The next day in the late afternoon, Sam & Michael come along, armed with a box of chocolates.

I put the tea on and let them all chat while I sit in the "goldfish bowl," writing. An hour later I get a call for more tea. When I go in, I can tell they are all enjoying the chocolates. Half the top row has been consumed. I mention to Mum to go easy on them, since too much sugar will affect her diabetes. They are all three laughing and generally having a good time, catching up with who was at the party and what a nice time they had. We thank them for bringing a most expensive magnum of champagne. After another hour or so, they have to leave and I return to take out the cups. As I walk in, Mum is in the process of consuming another chocolate. I exclaim, "Wow! You guys must like this chocolate." The whole top layer is gone.

Michael replies that he never eats the stuff; Sam says she is watching her weight, so she wouldn't eat any. "You mean Mum just ate the whole top of the box?" Mum's eyes open wide and she looks defiant! I *better* make this fast, I thought! She leans and reaches out for the box, I move forward quickly making a grab for the rest of the chocolates, I get there first, not responding to her loud protests as I do so. (I'll put them in the kitchen cupboard with the other treats. I know that the DNs will be able to check her blood level tomorrow morning as long as nothing happens in the meantime. I'll call the nurse tonight if I need to.)

The hugs and thanks are sweet and Sam states they will call or stop by again soon. It isn't long before Mum's temperature soars. Directing a fan on her and giving her ample water seems to work all right. I check on her throughout the night (I'm quite sure she has reached her sugar limit with the Chocolates).

When the DNs arrive in the morning, I explain about Mum's chocolate binge straight away. After they take the usual blood sample, they raise their eyebrows staring at the reading, alarmed, but not saying anything. They increase the medication dosage by a considerable amount to bring Mum's sugar levels back to some semblance of normality. They nicely and delicately advise Mum that she will likely put herself into a COMA if she eats that much chocolate again. (At least I don't look like the bad guy this time.) She doesn't like the thought of a coma, and offers to be good. She acknowledges though, that these are one of her favorite brands of chocolates and that they were nice going down. They all have a good chuckle, and proceed with their normal activities. The sheets have to be changed again this morning. They are soaking wet from last night's perspiration.

It is today that DNs notice indications of bedsores, even though this special airwave mattress is supposed to prevent them from occurring. The nurse suggests a unique combination of oil and cream for Mum's heels, elbows and any other pressure points in contact with the bed. Protective sheepskin wool pads are placed on the bed sheet and positioned under her rear cheeks to help prevent further skin damage.

This is a disappointing moment for Mum as she has hoped to avoid bedsores. The sling lifting process has also to be adjusted, to avoid putting pressure on these specific points. The nurse sprays the affected areas with a sticky film which, after drying, looks and acts like a thin, clear layer of skin; an additional aid to try to prevent further damage.

This is all quite a process and Mum has to lie quite still, without tilting her bed up and down too much, so as not to put pressure on the damaged areas.

Another of Mum's friends, Mary, starts to come over and rub Mum's arm in the late afternoons. Often she just sits and keeps her company. This allows me time to go shopping. Mum calls my cell phone often while I am out. I think is for reassurance and just to chitchat. I paint a picture of where I am, describing the food area and what is on display in the store I am in at the time. I also ask for her input on vegetables or other items I am about to buy. Doing this enables her to feel like she is participating in the shopping outing, allowing her to feel as if she is in the familiar places she used to so often frequent herself.

I like to do this. I make suggestions that make her laugh about food items I am just about to order, loud enough for her to hear: "Excuse me, sir. Can I have two pounds of the choicest… prawn legs, and make those peeled, please?" or "I like those carrots, do they come in another color?" and "Exactly how fresh are these eggs, are they boiled or fried and where do you keep the chickens?"

Although she can't concentrate for long, she still has the desire to view magazines and newspapers. So, when asked, I go over to the magazine rack, stand there and describe magazines on the shelf, telling her the headlines, and then buy a couple of the ones she likes the sound of.

It will soon be time for Mum to have a few days' rest in a luxury purpose-built care facility. They specialize in short term stays for homebound and terminally sick patients.

Apart from having become "tea boy," I am the official "carer" for Mum. Without me there, she would be under constant supervision and costing the government a not-so-small fortune. Consequently, the authorities see that there's wisdom in offering me a short break to recuperate, so that I can continue helping Mum in the long-term and government resources don't get drained. It is a good system and works well in this particular scenario.

The nursing home and I coordinate the events and care Mum needs from Friday morning to Monday afternoon, so that we can be sure she will be taken care of as well as possible. They are a kind and compassionate group of staff and volunteers, dedicated to making people in such circumstances as Mum's feel welcome, cared for and valued. If possible, they will cater to any need she has.

They have an amazing wheelchair that has a full body-length, continuous-air-ripple reclining seat and mattress system. It looks nicer than my car. A patient can recline in this chair for quite some time and, the most important consideration for Mum by far, one is able to push the patient out amongst the well-kept garden grounds of this facility. On a good day, a patient can be wheeled around the grounds and enjoy the beauty, and then be left in a shaded spot under a tree to relax alone -if desired- to view the lush beauty around and breathe in the fresh clean air. Well, that's what we have heard. I have planned to take a trip to London to stay with friends and see my cousins this weekend. I'll be leaving early Saturday morning.

Friday has come along already and I know that Mum is feeling apprehensive, but will be fine when she gets there. My sister and close friends have already arranged to stop by and see her over the weekend. An ambulance from the home arrives to pick her up. She is ready. I have packed enough personal belongings for her few days' stay. We kiss and hug our goodbyes. I'll let her get settled in and will stop by this afternoon before I prepare for my London trip. The ambulance pulls away as I close the front door. It is silent. I decide that I feel like having a five-minute rest and lie down. I wake up nearly three hours later. That feels so good!

As I arrive at the home mid-afternoon, I realize I've had a picture in my mind of how this place might look. It far exceeds my expectations! It is a beautiful old building that was originally built for retiring clergy as a retreat in which they might spend their last days. It is quite majestic and welcoming. I am directed to Mum, who is indeed outside having tea on the patio with friends, Laura and Adrian.

I order an extra tea for myself, and someone else makes it for a change. It becomes clear that Mum has not yet been for a push around the gardens. Apparently, one of the volunteers did try earlier but, as she arrived at an incline at the beginning of the walk,

153

she got stuck. The chair is quite big and very heavy, resembling a bed in the reclined sitting position, with wheels and handle brakes.

Mum indicates that she wants me to take her to find the big shaded tree area with the view. We get underway. It is indeed heavy at first, but once we get going, it glides along the path quite smoothly, as the sun shines through the trees on the right. She makes many comments about the flowers on either side of the path; she reaches back to touch my hand as she cries, saying, "Thank you for this. This is so beautiful."

In the distance there is the big tree where one can stop and just rest. Looking back, you can't see the patio area for the trees and lush green hedges. I position Mum under the tree as she desires, with the best view of the lawns and flowerbeds.

This is so nice for her. We sit in silence for a few moments. I sit on the bench, close my eyes, and lean back. Mum says, "Thank goodness! I really needed one of these." I take in a deep breath of fresh air agreeing, "Oh yeah. Me too!" I then start coughing as a thick cloud of unexpected cigarette smoke drifts over. Gasping, I reposition myself quickly upwind of her.

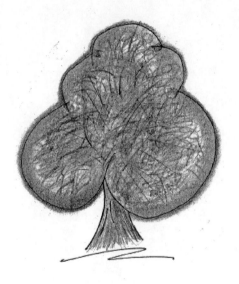

~ ✦ ~

Chapter 15

Three months have gone, I have to make plans.

Three months have already passed. If the doctors are right, only about three remain. I decide I ought to think about final preparations now rather than wait until after the event, when I will probably not be in the clearest state of mind. Crisis times are not the best to be making important decisions. I advise my sister about all that is going on, and ask her if she will help me after all the preliminary running around and sorting is done. I decide while I can to move forward and make as many of the arrangements in advance as are possible. I hope that there will be no decisions left to be made when the time comes, and we can just follow the arrangements as set.

I call, ask some questions and get prices from some local funeral services to give myself an idea of what's involved, but I am soon talking to some people much closer to home. I have known for a while that Mum's next door neighbors have a unique funeral service business. They organize traditional or "green burials." For "green burials," typically, the coffin is made of unfinished materials, which are strong and durable initially but biodegradable once in the ground. The final resting place is an area where, instead of traditional heavy gravestones being placed among a sea of others, a tree is planted instead, and a smaller stone plaque is placed securely on the grave.

Mum's friends are fully aware of the situation and are able to give me a few options to consider. One Saturday, while the pasty eater keeps watch, I tell Mum I will be going with some friends for a drive. They take me around some areas of Bristol to see some traditional overcrowded graveyards and then to view a "green site," which is just outside the city. It doesn't take long to figure out that the green location is the nicest. What a strange sensation I feel inside, doing this, but it has to be done. It feels both sad and hard to imagine that I won't be seeing my mum for much longer. Yet there is a peace that comes from doing what I am doing. I don't want a stranger figuring all this out. I want to be involved. I know my Mum, and I know what she would wish. The area is quiet, in the country, on a hillside overlooking other lush green areas of spacious farmland, with the sound of birdsong in the air. This is the place.

I collect brochures with pictures. What they depict, looking from an aerial perspective, is a cluster of three buildings in the south and immediately to the north. East and west are large areas of wooded and clear green pastured grounds, encompassing about 90 acres. We are looking at the clear green area on a hillside, just north of the northernmost building. The first structure is a beautifully refurbished farm complex, converted into a very large reception area. West of this is a chapel-like building, simple but peaceful, with tall double doors opening into a foyer area. A second set of doors opens into a white-walled open room, with plenty of seating in individual brown wooden chairs, divided by an aisle down the middle and with big windows high above on each side. It is all very light, airy and warm. This is a converted barn and is the place where the ceremonies are held.

Then, south of the farmhouse, is the cottage home of the keeper of the grounds. In between these buildings gray flagstones form a wide pathway which sweeps around, touching the front of all the buildings. In the center and surrounded by these same buildings is a lawn and a large pond. It is so picturesque that weddings are also celebrated here. I find all of this to be very uplifting, rather than the opposite! In my heart, I know this will be just right. I can see it as Mum's final resting place. I feel a big lump in my throat as I come to that decision. I take a brochure and, at the right time, I will show it to Mum. I will need to be sure she will like the idea and then do a follow up visit with my sister, so she can participate in choosing a specific site.

It is a quiet day with Mum. I bring her a fresh tea. I sit with my cup and then say, "Mum, what are your thoughts regarding final arrangements?" "I don't want to be cremated. I would like to be buried in a nice area. I don't want an open casket thing either. I do want to have my nice bright gown on." She indicated positively. "Well, I think my thoughts are along the same lines as yours. I knew you didn't want cremation, and I got the opportunity last week to visit a couple of places. I found one I thought you would like. Here is a picture of it." I proceed to describe the area further. "That sounds lovely, Lee. And tell everyone not to wear black! This is a celebration of my life, not a time for commiseration! Tell them to have a party after! What about music?" She smiled enthusiastically. "Do you have anything particular in mind?" I wondered. Yeah she beamed, how about "Andrea Bocelli - "Sagamo"- and the soft mix; then the Buddha party mix after!" "Alright then, I chimed. That will all be arranged. I hope you don't mind me getting this done in advance and if a miracle happens in the meantime, I can cancel it all."

I think it would be a tall order to arrange things at the last moment, especially when I can plan ahead.

"I'm glad you could have a say-so, Mum." "Yeah me, too. Any more tea, Lee?" "Yes, of course!"

As well meaning as she is about the party part, none of us will be quite in that mood at the time, I'm sure. (Although that *is* the normal custom for some)

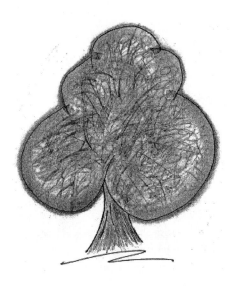

Chapter 16

Giving our permission

During these, her last three weeks, Mum has also been feeling pains in her abdomen, and is evidently fully aware of her path at this time. This is at no time clearer than when, one evening, after all has been said and done, she says, "What is the point?! What is the point of just lying here? There is nothing more for me. There is no quality of life! All I am doing is just lying here day in, day out…waiting to die. I'm tired of it, Lee. I'm tired of this existence." I stroke her head, and say, "I understand. All considered, you have done well to this point. You have had all your final wishes fulfilled." We reflect on her gatherings of friends, and finally the bonus time we have had together here as the result of this final illness. With all the courage and conviction I can muster from inside, I say, "Mum, you have done all you can do. Jasmine and I will be all right. There is nothing more for you to do here on this earth. We don't want you to have to continue in pain and suffer in this way any longer. You can let go whenever you are ready. You have our permission to leave, Mum, because we love you so much."

We both shed tears and hug. I understand what she means, and I know most people would at some point feel the same way. Mum's time has come. She is ready to complete the cycle of her life.

She seems more and more at peace, even though some days and nights are interrupted with the need for more pain-reducing medication. Mum says she will opt for a pump only when the pain starts becoming unbearable. The strong medication will come from a morphine pump, which has a fine tube going directly into a blood vessel. It has a hallucinogenic side effect, and she doesn't want to lose her sense of what is happening or for others to see her in a fuzzy minded state.

We talk about it and agree that when that level of pain arrives, I will be here, will watch all that happens and will take care of all that I can. "I won't leave. I'll be right here," I promise her. She accepts this and is at rest with the decision.

One morning when she is not in pain and has not needed medication the night before, she asks me, "Do you see the light? There is a glow in the room. Do you see it?" She notices my hesitation and assures me there's no need to be afraid, it is a good presence in this room. She says, "It's peaceful in here. Lee, He is still there, stroking my head and shoulder... I can feel it as soon as I close my eyes." She beams a wonderful smile.

The next few days and nights are not the easiest. She frequently wakes up during the night in pain, or not feeling well. Her appetite has diminished greatly, and she sleeps a lot more during the day.

After another few days her pain and discomfort increase to the point that, on the morning of June eighth after a particularly uncomfortable night, I ask her whether it is time. She holds my hand and says softly, "Yes, I think it is."

No more pain from today

I contact the DN, who comes within the hour bringing relief in a syringe pump not much bigger than a cell phone. She caringly connects the tiny tubes and supply, calculates the medications Mum has received, and sets the medication flow accordingly. The effect is swift. Mum enters into a deep sleep, and all other medications are stopped at this point.

The carers deal with her bedside needs without the lift system, as they have done these last few days. June eighth is a long day. Mum hardly has an appetite. In the afternoon, just in case she has a taste for something, I make her favorite dessert - semolina pudding. I mention it is available and her eyes open and light up. It is so good to give her something that she loves and eats! She is quiet, and has a sweet but helpless smile. Inside I'm crushed for her, but happy for the absence of pain. She finishes a few spoonfuls and gently leans back resting. I feel the need to call my sister, and a few of Mum's close friends, to indicate that her time is near. Perhaps a few days, one of the nurses suggests, or a week?

I know Mum's tender heart so well, and I think I understand how she feels at this time. I sit at the kitchen table and put my thoughts into words...

"Take me home"

Let the days get shorter. Oh let my days
go no longer. Do you hear me Lord?
I am ready for you, my Lord. Take me as I am.
My heart is open to you, my Lord. Take me as I am.
For to stay here paralyzed in bed in pain
Offers nothing more for me to gain.

Take me home, Lord, take me home...

I think of all the places I've been,
the sadness, but also the many joys I've seen.
The road has been long and steep at times;
but the love given and received got me through.
Just when I think it is all too much to bear
Your love, Lord, soothes just like warm air.

I have said goodbye to all those that I love.
I have shared my heart with those that would listen.
My soul now, like a dove, is ready to be free.

To those that I somehow forgot, you know me-
an elephant's memory I have not!

Take me home, Lord, take me home...

I hope GOOD memories of me
Will stay around, like an old oak tree.
Happiness, adventure and laughter galore;
for life around me was never a bore.
I have done what I've done and have said what I've said;
It has all brought me here to this place, in my bed.

Thank You for all of Your Love and for all of Your Prayers;
I will sleep now, and wait for the Lord to take me upstairs.
I long for the warmth of His eternal light;
For I am ready to come home.
With all my love, I wish you all...goodnight.

I'm coming home, Lord, I'm coming home.

164

~ ⚓ ~

The last time I say, "I love you."

Two good friends, Marianne and her daughter Savannah, feel a particular need to be close to Mum at this time, and come up from southern England. They arrive late on Sunday morning – June the ninth. Mum is mostly sleeping. By the afternoon, she wakes for just a little while and she asks for forgiveness of anything she may have said or done. I let the friends spend a little while with her. They try to hide their tears as well as they can, for Mum's sake. Mum seems to go in and out of a fuzzy Zone.

I have been sitting in the kitchen the last few moments when she calls my name loudly and purposefully: "Lee! Lee!" I jump up and, in a stride or two, I am there. "Yes, Mum...what is it?" I ask anxiously. She leans forward, reaches out her right hand and softly, but purposefully, clasps mine. With a loving smile and kindness in her eyes, looking straight at me, she says, "Lee, thank you, for everything. Thank you for all you've done. Thank you...I love you!" I gaze back into her eyes. "I love you, too, Mum." Tears well up in my eyes as the two friends stand quietly, tears streaming down their cheeks. Mum slowly lies back, closes her eyes and goes to sleep. We leave the room and stand in the kitchen. I hug them tightly as they cry and cry. We just stand like that for five minutes or so.

Time is moving, and they soon leave for the long trek back home. I am tired at this point, having had little sleep during the last four days and nights. I have been up for almost forty-eight hours. The DN, having been over late that day to check everything, orders a night relief nurse for the evening of June 9th, tonight and the next few nights, to enable me to sleep.

The carers come. There is not much to do again today, but to carefully empty the catheter bag and then leave.

Mum's lamp is glowing softly in the corner as the evening grows darker. I call Jasmine and repeat the news from the nurse, that perhaps a few days or a week are all the time Mum has. She says she will be over first thing in the morning. As the evening slowly wears on, I begin to feel utterly exhausted. Mum's friend, Natasha, stops by, enabling me to sit back and relax knowing another pair of eyes and ears are present. We have tea and chat about the day's events here with Mum, then have a light supper.

The night nurse arrives at 8:00 p.m. I settle her in and show her all she needs to know. She and Natasha chat for a while, but I can no longer keep my eyes open and retire to bed. I stay dressed, in case I am needed, dropping into a deep sleep as soon as my head touches the pillow.

~ ✦ ~

Her journey is underway

I am startled when the night nurse wakes me suddenly. "You'd better come in to see her right now!" In a moment I am kneeling by the bed, holding Mum's hand.

She then breathes out her last breath. I am silent, stunned. I look at the clock. It is 03:06 a.m. The little boy in me calls out, "Mum! Mum!" I put her still warm right hand next to my face and cry. I cry for her suffering during this time. I cry for the relief she has now found. I cry for the loss of my mum. I cry because I am thankful she is now in a better place. I cry because I will miss her so much...

The night nurse, in the meantime, goes to the kitchen and makes the calls notifying her network and the night doctor. I stay kneeling, leaning my face on her hand and taking deep breaths to calm down as I reflect on this moment in my life. A firm hand presses my shoulder. It's Natasha's - she hasn't left. I can't talk. There is nothing to say. I just stay right here, holding Mum's hand.

Natasha lights some candles, which cast a beautiful warm glow around the room. After twenty minutes or so, she and the night nurse stand, one each side of me, and slowly lift me to my feet. I stand to one side as they straighten Mum's bedcovers and pillows, and tuck her in. Mum looks so peaceful with a soft smile. I move over to the stereo and put on her favorite gentle music CD. It is so calm and peaceful. It is almost perfect.

167

We three sit in the kitchen hardly saying a word. The girls make tea. The nurse indicates that a night doctor will be calling in soon. Sure enough, at 04:30 a.m., in comes the doctor. She is softly-spoken and doesn't take much time to confirm that Mum has moved on from this life. There is no need for an ambulance. The local doctor will be here first thing at 08:00 a.m. to make the official pronouncement and provide the relevant papers. The night nurse and Natasha debate who will stay the rest of the night and they advise me to go lie down for a while, as all is in good hands. I think to call my sister but, at 04:42 a.m., I can wait a little longer, and call closer to her waking time. There is no rush, now. It will be busy these next few days so, indeed, I had best rest my head while I can.

~ ✦ ~

It's time to tell Jas

I wake up at 06:30 a.m., not sure if it's all just been a bad dream, as I hear a light knock on the door. "Lee, here's some tea!" It's Natasha. Bless her heart! She decided to stay around because she had sensed that Mum's time was close. She had recently cared for her own dad under similar circumstances, and recognized the signs. So she made arrangements for her mum to look after her daughter last night. It is time to call Jas. Mike picks up the phone first. He knows what's happened when he hears the tone of my voice. I go over the details so he is prepared to help comfort Jas. He passes the phone over and, as gently as I can, I break the news to my sister. The quiet sobs don't hide the pain she feels inside. I know Mike will give her the comfort she needs at this time. I hang up and think of the other people I need to call, and the rest of the

168

things to be done. I am relieved that the arrangements for her resting place have already been made. I thank Natasha for all she has done and for being such a good friend to Mum, and now to me too. She has to get going, and needs a good sleep herself as well. I clear up and start to prepare for the day. I restart the soft music as Mum lies peacefully. She will remain so for most of the morning until my sister arrives. I begin calling Mum's closest friends, and then leave a message for the funeral director.

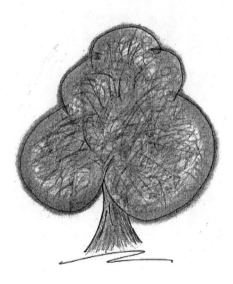

At 08:00 a.m. sharp the doctor comes, along with an assistant. He is from Mum's local doctors' office. He has to ask me a few standard questions and is very tender in his approach as he goes about the business of checking for vital signs. How gentle he is in making the official pronouncement! He gives me some official declaration papers that he has just signed and leaves shortly thereafter, just before the DN arrives with a couple of assistants. We have all become pretty close over the last six months. Mum was obviously somebody quite special to them, as they each became fond of her too. Although medical professionals do this sort of thing all the time, they naturally get a soft spot for certain people in particular. The fact that they were all so sweet to Mum made the whole time easier for her as well.

The calls come back pretty quickly. I am a little overwhelmed at first, but there is much to organize and I have to pull myself together and get on with it. I feel as if I am operating on "autopilot." I can manage from moment to moment, but I can't think back much further than this morning. I continue to call Mum's sisters, and a few others who were near and dear.

At about 10:30 a.m. Jasmine and Mike arrive, their eyes puffy and red. We comfort one another, then they enter into the peaceful room to sit with Mum.

~ ⚓ ~

The transport car arrives

Around 11:30 a.m., the funeral car comes to the back door to transport Mum to a holding area until all the final arrangements and protocol have been settled. I help maneuver the apparatus to make it easier for them to move Mum. Opening the closet, I pull out Mum's chosen colorful outfit, which puts a smile on my face. I give it to Mum's friend, the funeral director. It is quite quiet, as the music softly plays in the background. The undertakers finally position Mum onto the cart to wheel her away. I stand by and take one final opportunity to lean down and kiss her forehead. Jas hangs on to Mike, crying uncontrollably, as they start to move Mum slowly out of the room. I stand there alone and tremble with tears streaming down my cheeks.

This is the last time I will ever physically see Mum. I watch as they all walk outside. Just as they are about to place her in the vehicle, my sister cries out, "Let me see Mum! Wait! Let me see Mum again!" She runs out of the kitchen to kiss Mum, just one more time. Mum's friend comes back inside, tearful, and hugs me tightly. I just can't say anything.

She has to leave with the car and the best I can manage is a knowing nod of my head, understanding that it is time. The engine starts and through the window I can see the car slowly move off. The back door closes as Jas and Mike come in. We three sit in silence. It is time for "tea boy" once again to do his part. I wipe away my tears, and put the kettle on. Jasmine wants to know the events of last night, so I recite all that I can remember at this point.

I explain all that happened the previous day and looking back, Mum never woke up since that time she settled back into her pillows - after saying those few words to me. So she passed away peacefully in her sleep. We are glad of that, at least. It will be a few days before the burial. We decide that today we will simply tidy up a little and leave. I give the neighbors my cell phone number, grab a few belongings, close the door and ride home with Jas and Mike. I don't want to be alone tonight, and tomorrow will be another day. I can work on the official things then. For now, though, all I can think about is sleep.

~ ⚓ ~

Organizing the final events

After a few days of sorting and sending certificates, notifying official offices about Mum's passing and taking care of a few other administrative duties, the funeral date is confirmed. Jas and I each have a list of people to call, to advise them where and when the ceremony is to be held and to ask them not to wear black if at all possible. Phone calls and cards of love, flowers and warmth pour in over the next few days from England and the U.S. Lindsey, who is just like a granddaughter, calls to explain that she wants to contribute by providing the food and soft drinks for the gathering time after the service. She and her family provide a wonderful spread. Mum would have been so proud of her for doing this and, what's even more important, that she had the heart to think of making this contribution in the first place.

~ ⚜ ~

It is time. The day has arrived

It is a mild and somewhat overcast June day. A light breeze blows softly through the leaves, and the long green grasses in the meadows around are swaying with the changes of the wind. The chapel is full with a few family members, including Aunt Marion and Marco from London, as well as many friends, some of whom have traveled a very long way. Once again Natasha has worked her magic, with candles and flowers at the front of the Chapel and in the foyer.

Mum's soft instrumental music is playing. Most are dressed colorfully as requested, with a few feeling more comfortable in black. It is truly a special day.

The hearse arrives, and we meet it as it pulls up outside of the chapel. I am honored to be a bearer, with a few other strong men. We hoist the light-wooden coffin, which is knee tremblingly heavy, onto our shoulders. A lady gasps, as one of the chaps loses his footing when we start to move but thankfully catches himself.

We walk through the center of the chapel to the front, bringing the coffin to rest on a waist-high frame. The bearers leave, and I take my seat in the front. The music is turned off and the short service begins. Mum's dear friends, Laura and Adrian, are close to the front and Adrian opens the ceremony with a poem. He says a few words, by way of an introduction, thanking everybody for coming, and recognizing that each person present represents a life that Mum has touched, or is someone by whom Mum's life has been touched. In either case, we were all people very special to her. Adrian then invites me to step forward.

I proceed to read these words for Jas, Mandy and myself;

"Our Mum"

Our... mum what a special life, a diamond soul; what a presence of life!

She was not only a mum, she was also one of my truest and best friends. She did all she could, with what she had, to be a home mum. It wasn't perfect, we didn't have much growing up...but there was a lot of love and that made up for all the rest.

Mum was encouraging...throughout our childhood she would counsel strength, wisdom, honesty, love and compassion. She was always admired by friends. Good food and friends were a passion for her.

Growing up, our home was a busy home, always lots of people and friends coming and going. Some came for dinner, some came to get ingredients for their dinner. Many came for help and to be loved... some were sick and all were welcomed. Mum brought in people like some bring in stray pets – she was a surrogate mum to many. Good food, a hot drink, and a place to lay a weary head were options always offered. You never knew who was going to be sleeping in the front room.

Mum was a fighter throughout her life. Her own childhood was a mix of many challenges. She came through regardless of the tough odds. She had amazing internal fortitude and tenacity. This strength brought her through some of the toughest things life can throw.

She found a deeper happiness that she shared with all. As a child I recall many a trip to London to learn about a " knowledge within." Later she took on the faith of a Christian and enjoyed the praying, sharing, caring and love among them. Conversations with Mum as most know, were rarely on the surface. Our trip to India was one of the most memorable times in my life, sitting with swamis, yogis and mahatmas. It was quite a trip. From that time forward she became not just a mum, but a dear and cherished friend.

When the doctors could do no more for Mum, they had to let her go. There is peace in the acceptance that it's one's own time to go. Mum had this strength of peace...mentioned in the Bible as "a peace beyond all understanding." She is ready to move on to the vastness of eternity, the next journey into the soft eternal light.

174

I will reflect on the joy she brought into my life. Her laughter and smiles will be with me always, her love and devotion remembered and cherished. She made a huge difference in my life. I celebrate the life of our mum, Tina Hayward...she is no doubt soon going to be having a party somewhere in heaven, making new friends.

Mum, you are dearly loved and always remembered. Thank you for everything. We are so proud to say, "Tina Hayward, was our Mum!"

Adrian encourages others to come and say a few words if they feel led to do so. First Savannah steps forward, and sings a wonderful song in her beautiful voice repeating these words: "...and I will always love you, I will always love you, and I will always love you." A friend reads a few of his own words, affirming that Mum has been a great influence in his life. A few others share what's in their hearts. Adrian invites everyone to the actual laying to rest of the coffin.

As we all stand around, and before it is lowered, we hear birds singing nearby. As the coffin finally comes to rest, red roses are kissed and gently dropped in by family and close friends. I say a prayer.

We stand for quite a while in silence, lost in our own thoughts, in our remembrances. Tina was greatly loved and is already sorely missed. Slowly, some people begin meandering down the meadow towards the reception. Others stay on to reflect for a while longer.

~ ~

We gather and reflect

We all gather for delicious food, to enjoy gentle music and meeting friends. Stories are shared, of Mum's kindness, and her willingness to listen - she always gave generously of her time.

Others tell of fun times. Strangers introduce themselves to one another. It is yet another party Mum would have enjoyed herself. How strange, at funerals - the missing link is the person for whom everyone has gathered. Mum is the only one who would have known everyone here. But we all share in common a great regard for Mum. We all have a story to tell and we all loved her!

~ ~

As the green grass sways and birdsong fills the air, may the oak tree planted by Mum's graveside grow tall and strong, reaching to the sky. When Mum looks down from the Heavens, may she see her tree providing shelter and rest, stirring memories of good times shared with those friends who come by.

Love is never forgotten and so you remain in our hearts.

We enjoyed your "dash," Mum!

With much love

The end.

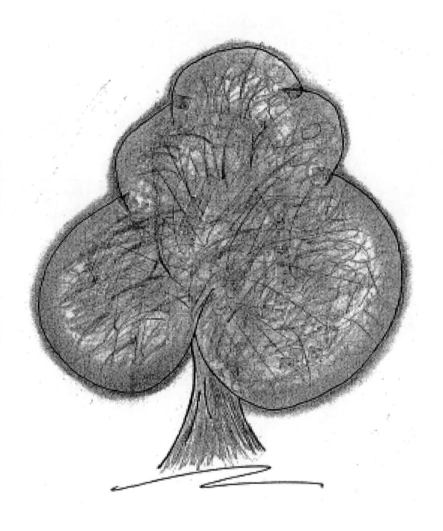

"The Oak tree"

Quick - chili beans on toast **A-lah-Mum**

<u>Ingredients:</u> (serves 4)
1 large can of baked beans.
1 large onion sliced thinly (not chopped and diced).
1 tablespoon of sugar.
2 tablespoons of Olive oil.
½ a teaspoon of chili powder, or 2 dried chilies for taste.

<u>Method:</u> (Have all ingredients ready and prepared) For the best results, cook slowly and clear up as you go.

Fry onions in oil till golden brown. Add contents of can. Add sugar and chili stirring it in. Then let it simmer for a good 10 minutes. (This should all be smelling good at about now.) Serve on golden brown toast.

Ready to devour. Enjoy the new taste. Enjoy the time with friends and family. Well, do you love it? *(A common question after mum dished out a meal)*

Tomato Breedy - Malaysian dish
(Best when cooked a day prior to eating)

Ingredients: (serves 4)

2 large cans of plum peeled tomatoes (no skin)
3 large onions (halved & sliced)
2 medium size potatoes (cut into quarters)
(with meat, use cut steak chunks and cook in with onions)
½ a teaspoon of chili
2 tablespoons of sugar
4 tablespoons of olive oil
3 thick sticks of cinnamon
Pinch of sea salt for taste

Method: (Have all ingredients ready and prepared) For the best results, cook slowly and clear up as you go.

Fry onions till golden brown. (Add meat now if used.) Add chili stir in and let cook for 1 minute. Add sugar, stir in well. Add cinnamon sticks stir in putting lid back on, let it cook in for a good 4 minutes. Add potatoes, stir in, add all tomatoes. Put on high for 20 minutes. Stir intermittently. Reduce to medium for another 20 minutes then take off from heat. Let it sit for another 10 minutes. Now ready to serve.

(The general "ready" indicator are the potato's, they should be soft enough for you to slide a fork through with ease.)

Rice:
Long grain rice
1 tablespoon of olive oil
4 cloves
½ a teaspoon of yellow tumeric

Method:

A medium size saucepan with lid.

Wash rice thoroughly. Let wet rice sit on side in a container.
Heat oil in pan, when hot enough add in all cloves, put lid on.
(don't burn the oil, turn down if need be) the cloves should soon
expand, you may hear them popping. Take off heat swirl them
around so that the oil takes on the clove scent. Now put the pan
back on the stove top, but OFF the heat. Open lid, now confidently
and quickly pour in all the wet rice, and then put the lid back on.
BE CAREFUL AS YOU DO, THE OIL WILL SPIT & MAKE A
NOISE. Once the noise has calmed down, open lid add water to
about ½ inch depth over rice, stir in the tumeric, now cook down
till rice is soft and ready to eat.

This meal is my personal favorite meal of all. I hope you enjoy it
as much as I still do. Enjoy the time with family and friends.

The Breedy is good too when served cold.

Drop me a line…and let me know if you "Love it!"

The Epilogue

I eventually returned to the U.S. at the beginning of November 2002. It was the end of a journey in one sense and the beginning of another in another!

So, where do we go from here? How do we go on with life now? Slowly... we just go very slowly.

Take time to know and feel your sorrow. Life will be different from now on. Christmas will be different: Special times and places will feel different. The process of grieving is so essential... it is alright to let yourself grieve, and it takes time – longer than our impatient society cares to admit or really understand. If possible, grieve with a close friend or relative. Allow others to give you comfort and resist the temptation to be an island all on your own if you can help it.

Hold on to the memories of the close bond you've shared. They will comfort you and will give you the lift and strength to make it through those difficult days. As a flowerbed in winter looks bare and unpromising yet is bursting with life in the spring, yours too will bloom again, my friend. Spring will surely come back into your life once again. It just takes time.

It's a mysterious process, one which we little understand, but somehow we are able to move on eventually, even if we start with just one small step to at a time. Have the faith and courage to go forward: "Now faith is the substance of things hoped for, the evidence of things not seen." Heb 11:1 (KJV)

Put the tea on!

Okay, now put the tea on ("English breakfast," of course!) At some moment when you feel ready, make a list of things to sort out. Here are some brief sketchy ideas to help you along. You'll inevitably think of others too - they'll vary with the situation and the place you currently stand in relation to an ill or terminal friend or relative. These suggestions are offered in no particular order of priority or importance, and you soon learn to discern which concerns can wait for attention and which cannot.

While dealing with the care of a close relative or friend who is terminally ill:

Planning ahead can be invaluable. Even some basic insurance coverage can take care of areas that might otherwise be a major concern when (not if) the event occurs. It made life much easier for me and my sister because we did make some plans before Mum began experiencing health problems. Take care of this and then put the papers away in a safe place and don't think about it anymore. I *strongly* encourage you to do this.

PLEASE NOTE: I am not a professional and am not giving advice in any official capacity, merely recounting my experiences and some lessons I learned that I feel might be helpful to others. I do counsel you to seek good professional advice.

It can't hurt to discuss your situation with a qualified financial advisor, insurance agent, accountant and attorney, to help you with areas in which you may not otherwise feel capable of making a decision. There will be final expenses to take into consideration, maybe a "Will" to initiate. If there is still time it certainly could pay to chat this over with an attorney – where there's money and property involved in a person's estate, sometimes creative planning can be really helpful. The laws regarding legacies are quite complicated. Practical concerns will weigh heavily on a dying person in many cases. It is surprising how people will hang on, often contrary to predictions of the medical people, until they are sure it's okay for them to "let go" and leave their affairs in the hands of people they trust to take care of their families, assets and business affairs in accordance with their deeply felt wishes. If something like a will has been left until the last minute, it may really help your patient to be able to relax and make the transition if you can help him or her to arrange to have one drawn up.

In the same way, making plans for the funeral and final resting place, any special requests concerning music, words to be spoken, sung, engraved and so on, can be very helpful to some people while others would be horrified at the thought of talking about anything other than full recovery. You have to feel it out, but probably have a good idea of your own loved one's psychological makeup and attitudes in this regard.

Whether or not it feels appropriate to discuss funeral and burial plans with the person for whom you're caring, it might well be helpful for you yourself to work out some ideas in advance. Otherwise you may find you're the person with all the organizing to do just at the time when you're emotionally shell-shocked by your own bereavement and feel least able to cope with this. No matter how long a death is anticipated it is always a terrible shock when it actually occurs, and you'd do well -if you have time and energy to make some preparations in this area- to cut yourself some slack at this critical time. You might even draft the large part of a letter to send out informing everyone, for when the time comes. Having an idea of timescales is also an important consideration. As time goes on and you grow more tired and strained yourself you will probably want to find out from the medical staff most closely involved what their expectations are at any given time. You will inevitably get progressively drained yourself during a long period of caring, and as the patient's condition and quite possibly spirits too deteriorate. It is essential that you try to work out how to pace yourself, in as much as possible. Doctors rarely like to predict anything with much certainty, as they might often be proved wrong if they were inclined to do so. It can be a case of having to read between the lines. In my personal experience nursing staff, who supervise care on a daily basis, can be more forthcoming and have a fairly accurate sense of the way things seem to be tending.

Take care throughout, of your own health and sanity first, anyhow (otherwise you're no help to anyone), and then of those near and dear. Comfort each other and understand there may be confusion and anger (there will often be mixed emotions), and that there is little time for reflection or resolution of all this at this time. There may well be at some point, when you can stop and everything becomes more balanced again.

Consider a visit and a chat with your local hospice organization. They have a variety of information that will help you. Breaks, as I mentioned, can be arranged both the patient and for the carer too, where required. There are also numerous leaflets, phone and internet help and information lines you can find out about through your library, doctor's office or local hospice organization.

Upon the person's passing away. Some purely practical thoughts:

After the death certificate [so called in England] is obtained, personal items like passports, driving licenses, social security and credit cards need to be cancelled, the relevant authorities notified. Have certified copies of the official death certificate handy to send out with official cancellations/notifications. Make up a standard generic letter to send out. Some agencies will require an original certified copy of the certificate while other organizations will be satisfied with only a photocopy. (Originals are usually returned to you.) There will be various banking considerations – for instance, the deceased's bank account will be "frozen" upon notification of the death. It can be useful to be aware of this fact as this can cause problems for the spouse. Get professional advice as to the advantages or disadvantages of adjusting the bank account into "joint" status. Direct debits and various insurances (including vehicle cover) need to be looked at, and any refunds applied for where applicable.

For a while, mail will still arrive in the person's name and calls too will be likely to come in for him or her. Often it will be an old friend, a work associate or perhaps a fellow member of an organization attended, each caller not having heard the news for some reason or other. Some people, blundering into this situation, simply don't know what to say - they don't mean to be insensitive but, ironically, you somehow end up having to be the one offering encouragement and comfort to them! Every time you have to explain the present circumstances… it's not easy. As time goes on such calls will diminish and you will adapt. Let those who really care about you nurture and encourage you now.

Understand that you are emotionally vulnerable at this point. Consequently any major or life-changing decisions ought to be postponed if possible, and new opportunities put to the side for the time being. Give yourself some time and space to think and re-group. Don't rush. "If in doubt, hesitate," I believe the saying goes! You owe it to yourself, and are entitled to this consideration.

Finally, whenever you can, make the time to be still and sit quietly. It is amazing the wisdom that can come to us as if by magic if we simply sit back and allow ourselves to know intuitively the best course of action, or inaction, at any given moment. Prayer time with close friends, too, can give some much-needed clarity concerning your new circumstances. It certainly was invaluable for me.

We would greatly appreciate your comments, please send them to:

e-mail: Sixmonthstosaygoodbye@yahoo.com

Or

write via the publisher: Lord and Ward Publishing
3837 Northdale Blvd #112
Tampa, FL 33624

www.lordandwardpublishing.com